Learning Re-enabled

A Practical Guide to Helping Children with Learning Disabilities

SECOND EDITION

SUSAN N. SCHRIBER ORLOFF, OTR/L

Executive Director,
Children's Special Services, LLC,
Atlanta, Georgia

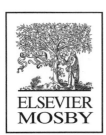

ELSEVIER
MOSBY

**ELSEVIER
MOSBY**

11830 Westline Industrial Drive
St. Louis, MO 63146

LEARNING RE-ENABLED: A PRACTICAL GUIDE TO HELPING CHILDREN   0-323-02772-5
WITH LEARNING DISABILITIES

NOTICE

Occupational therapy/special education is an ever-changing field. Standard safety precautions must be
followed, but as new research and clinical experience broaden our knowledge, changes in treatment
and drug therapy may become necessary or appropriate. Readers are advised to check the most current
product information provided by the manufacturer of each drug to be administered to verify the
recommended dose, the method and duration of administration, and contraindications. It is the
responsibility of the licensed prescriber, relying on experience and knowledge of the patient, to
determine dosages and the best treatment for each individual patient. Neither the publisher nor the
author assumes any liability for any injury and/or damage to persons or property arising from this
publication.

International Standard Book Number 0-323-02772-5

Publisher: Linda Duncan
Managing Editor: Kathryn Falk
Publishing Services Manager: Pat Joiner
Project Manager: Gena Magouirk
Design Project Manager: Bill Drone

Printed in USA.

Last digit is the print number: 9   8   7   6   5   4   3   2   1

In loving memory of my parents, Lillian Levinson Schriber and Max Schriber. Your lessons in life and love live on as a vibrant guide and a loving benediction.

Road, n.

A strip of land along which one may pass from
where it is too tiresome to be to where
it is futile to go.

Ambrose Bierce
U.S. Political Journalist
1842-1914(?)

And so this pessimistic view of life in the early part of
the last century seems very close to what some
children are probably feeling about their daily life in
school.

It is anxiety-provoking and tiresome to go to a place
every day where, no matter how hard you try – *you fail.*

WHY OT?
AND WHAT CAN IT DO AND NOT DO FOR YOUR NEEDS?

If you have ever asked yourself...
Why me?
Why my child?
How can this be?
Where do I go?
What does this mean?
Why didn't my pediatrician/doctor pick this up?
Where do I start?
Can this be fixed?

The possibility exists that if you are reading this book, you are either a parent, a teacher, a therapist, or an individual with a learning disability.

It is the mission of this book to talk with and to you. Irrespective of what you may feel inside, what kids on the playground have said, or a boss made you feel, YOU are not "damaged goods." We all have our unique style of doing things. If we were all the same, we would all be Einsteins, Olympic athletes, and world-renowned scientists. Where to go, what to do, how to do it, what to expect: It is the intent of our services to answer these key questions and to give you a foundation from which to be both an informed consumer and an advocate for yourself, your child, or your student.

Your reactions are normal, and they need to be addressed, acknowledged, and responded to with empathy and constructive support.

So if you have ever asked yourself: Why me? Why my child? How can this be? Where do I go? What does this mean? Why didn't my pediatrician/doctor pick this up? Where do I start? Can this be fixed?, you are not alone. This is often the first set of questions parents, children, and other "first-time hearers" ask themselves and anyone they feel they can trust or in whom they have placed educational confidence. The denial, the anger, and the need to control, if taken at face value, are obnoxious, distancing behaviors that impede rather than impel parents into proactive positive directions and, ultimately, solutions for their children's learning issues.

They are good questions. They are valid. However they are more than that. They are lifelines, not yet attached, not yet secured, which if allowed to tether properly, will serve to guide both the parent and the child into safer waters.

The parents must simultaneously learn the lingo, make discriminating choices, and trust at a time when they feel as if they have been transplanted to the proverbial shifting sands.

And then some matter-of-fact administrator, teacher, or psychologist plays Sergeant Friday and just "gives'em the facts,"and we well-intentioned professionals wonder in amazement just why these supposedly well-educated people are so weird!

It is from this vantage point that parents read the initial reports in unfamiliar lingo while sitting on unfamiliar shifting sands. Often on those reports the recommendation is to have an "occupational therapy" evaluation. More new words, more new people, more trusting what is foreign, more fear. Parents come into occupational therapy not knowing what to expect, protective of their child, half-hearing, whole-heartedly hoping this will "fix it."

Thus comes the second set of questions: How much? How often? It is a time of emotional free-fall for parent and child, and the job of guiding that flight often falls to the pediatric occupational therapist.

The careful application of sensory, integrative, cognitive, perceptual, and developmental therapies is the essence of individualized occupational therapy. The stuff parents and teachers see—coloring, cutting, drawing, building, playing, remembering—happen only after specific neurosensory developmental abilities have reached a level of meaningful processing. Ferreting out the difference between a resistive behavior and an unstable perceptual system of a child is the art of occupational therapy. Understanding the neuromuscular organic systems influencing these reactions is the science of occupational therapy. The therapeutic application of activity is the culmination of both the art (intuitive) and the science (factual) of play and class simulation in occupational therapy.

However, with the art and science must come the empathy. Both parent and child are entering a situation fraught with uncertainties. It is the job of the occupational therapist to calm the fears and make familiar that which is not.

No pediatric occupational therapy program can be successful without the comments and participation of the parents. They are the foundation from which we begin our work together. We all exist within the context in which we live—our homes, our families, our friends, our jobs. For children, their "job" is going to school. It is what they must do every day. For some children, just the act of entering the classroom can be overwhelming.

To manage fears, to find solutions, to expand choices, and to discover inner trust—these are the real goals of occupational therapy. When that happens, all the rest of the fabulous puzzle that is your child comes together.

ACKNOWLEDGMENTS

I would like to thank Chris Bonsonatta Doane, MS OTR/L, President of Advanced Rehabilitation Services, for her guidance and generosity. She let me participate in the development of her company, which specializes in staffing and continuing education.

Originally, my company, Children's Special Services, was a division of Advanced Rehabilitation Services. Upon Chris's insistence, we made Children's Special Services, LLC a separate entity. Chris, this book is a tribute to your support and confidence in me. Your wisdom and friendship continue to guide me, nurture me, and sustain me.

I also would like to recognize the support staff from Advanced Rehabilitation Services, Inc.: Teddi, Bobbi, Beth, and Lorraine. *Thank you* for always being there for me. You all are consistently supporting me, handling workshops, and assisting with staffing. To former ARS therapist, Pam Dillard, I wish to say a most sincere *thank you* for your patience with me as I learned how to run a business, pace clients, and mentor additional therapists. It has been a pleasure to be part of your professional and personal life.

To all the children with whom I have worked over the years, *thank you* for briefly letting me into your lives. A special *thank you* to all the children who came in on a sunny summer weekend morning so that the photos you see in this book could be taken. A very special *thank you* to Allison and Austin LaBreque, Kaitlin Mullen, Eric Campos, Andy Howell, and Phillip and Nathan Brown.

Thank you also to the many professionals and school principals and directors who had faith in me and allowed occupational therapy into their curricula when even the words seemed weird and out of place. To the faculties and staffs at the Heiskell School, Greenfield Hebrew Academy, The Schenk School, Woodward Academy, Mt. Vernon Presbyterian School, Eaton Learning Labs, Dunwoody Prep Pre-School, Kehelliat Chaim Pre-School, Infants of Dunwoody, the Epstein School, and the Davis Academy all in the Atlanta, Georgia area: *thank you* for helping me make my professional dreams come true.

This book would never have come to be without the guidance, corrections, interjections, creativity, enthusiasm, direction, and support of Kathy Falk, my editor, and Gena Magouirk, who proofread and fine tuned this manuscript.

And last but not least, to my children, Jenny, Rachel, and Nathan. Seeing their learning struggles through their eyes has allowed me to help other children with more clarity.

And to David, my husband and best friend, all of this is possible because you constantly support and sustain me.

TABLE OF CONTENTS

Introduction — Page 1

CHAPTER 1
Learning Disability in Plain English — Page 5

CHAPTER 2
What is Memory? — Page 19

CHAPTER 3
How We Learn — Page 23

CHAPTER 4
Piaget's Theories Simplified — Page 27

CHAPTER 5
Guidelines for Parents — Page 33

CHAPTER 6
Guidelines for Teachers — Page 71

CHAPTER 7
Occupational Therapy in Action — Page 85

CHAPTER 8
Student Writing Samples — Page 107

APPENDIX A
Function-based Glossary — Page 119

Page 139

APPENDIX B

What Does Uncle Sam Say About All of This?

APPENDIX C

Page 147

Section 504 Student Accommodation Plan

APPENDIX D

Page 149

Section 504 Parent Rights

APPENDIX E

Page 151

Classroom and Facility Accommodations

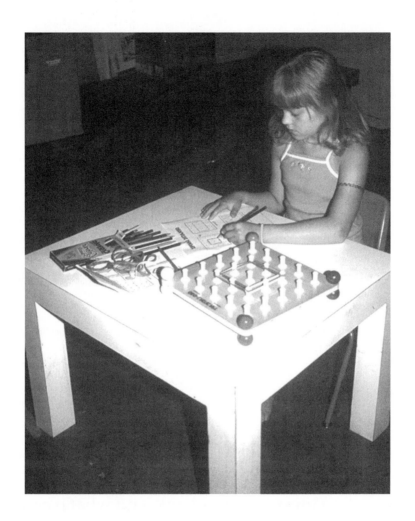

Introduction

This book is all about you, the Listener, the Hearer, the Sayer. Whether you are a teacher or a therapist or a parent, this is about COMMUNICATION.

How to say it.
How to ask it.
How to hear it.

There is no way to delete emotion. The information is hard to say, hard to hear, and hard to decipher.

To the parent:
This is **your kid**. No one knows him better.

To the teacher:
You know him thoroughly in task and in socially specific situations.

To the therapist:
This is the child you have looked at through the microscope of acumen; you've got his style nailed.

How can all these essential people coalesce proactively? How can they become cooperating citizens of this child's Babel when they all speak a different language from the heart? How in the world to reach accurate interpretations of all our crucial messages? So this book is about your needs, written by a former special education teacher, a parent of learning-disabled children, and a practicing occupational therapist.

How to use this book, and what it can (and cannot) do for you

This book is designed to help decipher the maze of information and the confusing, often pressured decisions that parents and teachers (as well as individuals themselves) feel when confronted with situations implying a learning disability.

This book is designed to answer your whats, whens, and hows: *What* is a learning disability? *What* is "normal development"? *When* should you pursue extended help? *How* can you go about getting help? *How* can you help your child at home?

It does not answer: Why you? Why your child? or Why did this happen? For those questions, there are no answers. As billions of cells combine and recombine as an individual is being formed before, at, and after birth, many of the combinations are a result of random pairings as well as those predetermined by genetics. This is no one's fault.

This book is not designed to help you diagnose your child. For that, you need specialized testing from an educational and developmental psychologist.

Chapters 1 to 4 describe what a learning disability is and is not. They illustrate how we learn and how we can adapt learning styles for success. Chapters 5 and 6 scope out developmental frameworks, what the "average" (whatever that means) individual is doing at a particular milestone, and what red flags to respond to or ignore. You are walked through the evaluation and IEP (individual education plan) processes. You will find a to-do suggestion box, suggested activities, and lists of learning toys and equipment and places to buy them. Pictorial demonstrations of occupational therapy in action and writing samples that show dramatic changes in writing skills after therapy are found in Chapters 7 and 8. Finally, in the Appendices you will find a glossary and even more information on the IDEA, Section 504 of the Rehabilitation Act of 1973, and the Americans with Disabilities Act.

Remember that there is no expert who will know more about your child than you do. The psychologist, the occupational therapist, and the teacher only see your child in short capsules of time in very specific situations. You, ultimately, are the one in charge. I have found over the years that the only mistake parents make (myself included) is thinking the issues will "grow away." The nagging feeling you have when your child is 3 or 4 can be quieted briefly, but it cannot disappear. Early intervention can help quell the anxiety for both you and your child.

I have written this book to be a conversation between us—parent to parent. I have been where you are. I have walked the walk, and I have talked the talk. I have been spoken to and told flat out: "Something is wrong with your child." I have had to find solutions. My children have all gone to college and are leading independent, successful lives. This book is to support you on this uncharted journey toward your personal solutions. Take a deep breath. You are not alone.

Notes
Take notes here and anywhere else. This is a working instructive book for you.

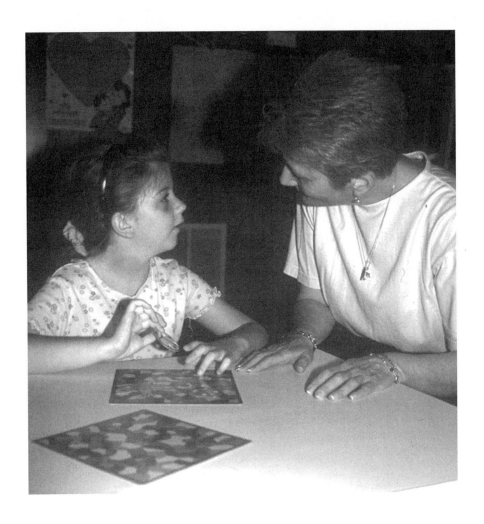

CHAPTER ONE

Learning Disability
in Plain English

Kids Who Are Different

Here's to the kids who are different.

The kids who don't always get A's.

The kids who have ears twice

The size of their peers',

And noses that go on for days . . .

Here's to the kids who are different.

The kids they call crazy or dumb.

The kids who don't fit,

With the guts and the grit,

Who dance to a different drum . . .

Here's to the kids who are different.

The kids with the mischievous streak.

For when they have grown,

As history's shown,

It's their difference that

Makes them unique.

Digby Wolfe

What is a Learning *Difference*?
What is a Learning *Disability*?

"Mr. and Mrs. Smith, John seems to have some developmental issues."

"I don't want my kid labeled! It might wind up in writing!"

And so the *dance* begins—an offbeat dance, with syncopated rhythms, in both major and minor chords.

Definitions in Plain English

Learning difference

Negative deviation from the "normal" learning style that appears to hamper the initiation and completion of activities or retention of needed information.

Learning disability (LD)

Difficulty in learning specific abilities or functions, while learning of other abilities or functions may be average or, in many cases, above average or superior.

IQ (intelligence quotient)

A specific measure of intelligence that is a composite of verbal and performance scores. Verbal scores reflect nonmotor skills, whereas performance scores reflect cognitive motor skills.

Attention deficit disorder

A description of behaviors that include difficulty attending, retaining, organizing, and producing specific tasks. This can sometimes, but not always, be accompanied by hyperactivity, which may be complicated by random, uncontrolled motor responses.

Graphomotor skills

Skills including planning and execution, with and without visual stimuli.

Handedness

Development of a dominant hand for writing and manipulation.

Muscle tone vs strength

Muscle tone is the ability to sustain co-construction in both dynamic and static modes; *strength* is force exerted on an object (the ability to use more than one muscle group to maintain a position).

Visual-motor skills

Ability to visually organize and associate visual stimuli.

Midline development

Development of skills that allow for focal manipulation at the center of the body with peripheral flow from the left to the right as needed for the development of reading and prereading skills.

Peripheral vs focal vision

Normally 80% of the average person's vision is peripheral; 20% is focal. Children with visual-perceptual problems usually have these percentages reversed.

Vestibular disorder

Difficulty in left/right coordination, eye movement, balance, and tactile interpretations. The vestibule is located in the semicircular canals and labyrinths of the ear. Under- or overreactions here can contribute to distorted sensory processing, which in turn can contribute to both behavioral and learning problems.

Some Common *Classroom* Signs of Discrete LD

1. Inattentiveness

2. Disorganization

3. Need for repeated instructions

4. Easy frustration

5. Slow work

6. Poor handwriting

7. Social problems (mild to moderate)

8. A child who seems very bright, but just isn't "getting it done"

Some Common *Home* Signs of Discrete LD

1. Problems with dressing and self-care beyond anticipated age of competency

2. Losing personal items

3. Forgetting familiar chores/homework

4. Difficulty with cooperative tasks

5. Difficulty with personal space

6. Oversensitivity with family members and friends

7. Rejecting or excessively fearing slightly familiar or unfamiliar situations

8. Few (new) friends

OCCUPATIONAL THERAPY DEFINITIONS
Scope of Occupational Therapy

Occupational therapy (OT) is a treatment that is medically based to provide both habilitation and rehabilitation to individuals experiencing difficulties in daily life functions. For children this includes, but is not limited to, assistance with the attainment of age-appropriate motor and visual-perceptual abilities.

School-Based Occupational Therapy

OT is a related support service that is initiated as an intervention after other traditional educational methods have failed. It must be based on educational goals and support objectives as written in the student's individual education plan (IEP).

Therapy duration and session length are decided by the IEP team (teacher, county representative, therapist, psychologist, school support services personnel, and parent).

Services can be either direct or indirect. *Direct services* (fine motor, perceptual-motor, sensory training, activities of daily living [ADLs], technological modifications, etc.) are usually provided in small groups, one-on-one with the student, or in inclusion class settings. Sometimes these services are directly delivered by a certified occupational therapy assistant (COTA) under the supervision of a registered occupational therapist (OTR).

Indirect services are usually consultative. The OTR consults with other educational staff (classroom teacher, resource teacher, educational specialists, etc.) about the student's special issues, needs, and concerns and provides suggestions for adaptations and/or modifications as needed. In this situation, the OTR may also meet with the student on a limited basis.

Private Occupational Therapy

Not restricted by the limits of an IEP, *private occupational therapy* can integrate all aspects of development: sensory, motor, visual, and emotional. Therapy duration and session length are determined collaboratively by both the parent and the therapist.

How Occupational Therapy Helps Learning	
0 to 18 Months **Reflex Reactions** Infant protective responses Survival mechanism 1	**19 to 36 Months** **Sensory Awareness** Touch Hot/cold perception Hearing Smell 2
36 Months to 5 Years **Neuro/Sensory Organization** Balance Perception Visual discrimination Fine motor manipulation Gross motor planning 3	**Functional End Products** Drawing Coloring Writing Numbers Graphs Reading Copying 4

Sensory Integration

Sensory integration is the ability of the brain to receive, interpret, and act upon accurate incoming information to produce desired cognitive-motor responses. The elements of sensory integration are:

Occupational therapy addresses boxes 1, 2, and 3, so that the "stuff" of school, box 4, becomes much easier.

Don't be put off by the lingo. This is what we all do everyday without thinking about it.

Proprioception

Muscle-bone-joint awareness; the ability to know what position your body is in without seeing it.

Kinesthesia

An internal map that lets you know which direction to go and how to move.

Diadochokensia

Communication across the two hemispheres of the brain that are responsible for right/left coordination.

Body position in space

The ability to know "which end is up."

Tactile perception

The ability to know if you are being touched and to discern what you are touching, as well as the pressure and intensity.

Localization of tactile stimuli

The ability to know where you are being touched.

Vestibular responses

Inner ear balance mechanisms that also coordinate the eyes and allow for crossing the midline.

Auditory perception

The ability to distinguish sounds.

Localization of auditory stimuli

The ability to tell where sounds are coming from.

Auditory defensiveness

A defensive response to noxious sound.

Auditory confusion

An inability to discriminate and isolate sounds in the presence of distracting background noises.

Gross Motor vs Fine Motor Movements

Gross motor movements

Large muscle movements that primarily contribute to mobility and stability patterns as well as ambulation and gross postural adjustments.

Fine motor movements

Small muscle movements that control dexterity including the refined movements of the hands, tongue, eyes, and toes, as well as discrete postural adjustments.

Visual Perception

Visual perception is the brain's ability to receive, interpret, and act upon visual stimuli. Perception is based on the following seven elements:

1. **Visual discrimination**
   The ability to distinguish one shape from another.

2. **Visual memory**
   The ability to remember a specific form when removed from your visual field.

3. **Visual-spatial relationships**
   The ability to recognize forms that are the same but may be in a different spatial orientation.

4. **Visual form constancy**
   The ability to discern similar forms that may be different in size, color, or spatial orientation and to consistently match the similar forms.

5. **Visual sequential memory**
   The ability to recall two to seven items in sequence with vision occluded.

6. **Visual figure/ground**
   The ability to discern discrete forms when camouflaged or partially hidden.

7. **Visual closure**
   The ability to recognize familiar forms that are only partially completed.

N o t e s

Read first, and then list the concerns you have about your child.

N o t e s

What is an Occupational Therapy Evaluation?

An OT program is designed after a complex evaluation. Many tools are used for the evaluation. Some are standardized, meaning they are scored on a statistical standard. Some are criterion-referenced, meaning performances are judged on an average performance scale for a specific age group. Others are clinical observations; the OTR looks at the style and form with which the child does specific tasks.

How long is an evaluation?

Because each therapist and clinic varies, ask before the test date how long the evaluation takes, how much the evaluation costs, and if you can observe.

How long is the course of therapy?

Again, the length of therapy is dependent upon the problems found. It is important for parents to ask their provider what the average length of treatment is. Treatment is usually once a week for 50 minutes. Depending upon the school, many private schools allow Children's Special Services, LLC, to come into the school and provide services on site. Ask your therapist and school about this.

Explanation of Standardized Tests

ETCH

The evaluations described here, like many other generalizations, are unique to this author's company, Children's Special Services. When seeking an occupational therapy evaluation, ask beforehand what tools the company uses.

For the most part, you can find samples of these on the internet: www.aota.org

The ETCH is a standardized test of handwriting performance that evaluates legibility, size, formation, writing line awareness, spacing, and sequencing. A score of 95% is considered fluid writing. Included in the test samples are near- and far-point copy skills as well as dictation and number writing.

Neurofunctional assessment

The neurofunctional assessment tests how the child approaches, executes, and completes specific developmental tasks. This assessment of neuromotor abilities tests the child's functional responses in play/game situations. It factors visual, sensory, motor, and cognitive components of a task. A comprehensive neurofunctional assessment should include the following items in a standard testing format: reaching patterns, grasp-release hand functions, balance and vibratory responses, tactile discrimination, etc. These are sometimes called *clinical observations*.

Goodenough-Harris Drawing Test

The Goodenough-Harris Drawing Test is a test of fine motor-cognitive-organizational abilities as well as body image.

PEER

The Pediatric Evaluation of Educational Readiness (PEER) is a multitask evaluation that combines neurodevelopmental, behavioral, and health components. It provides normative scored observations that help define developmental areas of concern. It evaluates developmental attainment, associated observation, and neuromaturation, as well as a task analysis of the input (visual, verbal, sequential, and somesthetic), storage (short-term memory and experiential acquisition), and output (fine motor, motor sequence, verbal sequence, and verbal expressive) functions.

Visual-motor inventory

The visual-motor inventory (VMI) and the subtests for visual perception and motor abilities are standardized tests that evaluate both the visual-motor abilities and the visual *and* motor abilities in isolation. These tests are used to help identify significant difficulties in the areas of coordination and perceptual-motor and -nonmotor integration.

Wide-range assessment of visual-motor abilities

The wide-range assessment of visual-motor abilities (WRAVMA) tests the child in the three spheres of visual-motor/perceptual development. It provides a psychometrically sound assessment of visual-motor, visual-spatial, and fine motor skills. A score of 100 (50%) out of a possible 200 is within the average range (98-103).

Test of visual-perceptual skills (nonmotor)

The test of visual-perceptual skills (TVPS) (nonmotor) assesses all of the same areas as the VMI, with the exception of the motor component. Thus it is able to distinguish between perception skills and motor skills. It is these discrete visual-perceptual abilities that are essential for comprehensive, organized, receptive, and expressive motor production.

Handwriting Without Tears evaluation

The Handwriting Without Tears evaluation is a criterion-referenced test of paper/pencil production that looks at habituated responses from memory and with a sample.

Sensory modulation/regulation assessment

The sensory modulation/regulation assessment looks at the tactile, visual, proprioceptive, vestibular, auditory, taste/oral, and olfactory sensory systems, observing both attentional and regulatory responses.

OT "play/sensory" evaluation

The OT "play/sensory" evaluation looks at approach, language, and behavior in various novel motor tasks.

Notes

The Essence of Occupational Therapy

Occupational therapy addresses all the items listed here to reconstruct the neuromotor, psychosocial foundations of development and learning so that the functional results will be commensurate with the desired outcomes, producing both an intellectual and an emotionally gratifying experience.

N o t e s

How does your child express his
"sensory self"?

Sensory History

Sensory History is a standardized checklist formulated by Winnie Dunn, OTR for the purpose of determining which situations elicit overly alert behavioral responses. It covers auditory, visual, tactile, movement, body position, emotional/social, and activity level responses. Its scores are *always, frequently, occasionally, seldom,* and *never*.

Behaviors

Vision

Tracking
Convergence
Quick localization

Reaching Patterns and Grasp-Release Patterns

Bimanual functions
    Cutting
    Reaching for a ball (with and without two hands)
Rapid forearm rotations (diadochokinesia)
Isolated finger control
Strength and range of motion
Muscle tone
Equilibrium
Upper extremity stability / weight shift

Reflexes

Protective reactions
ATNR/STNR
Schilders arm extension
    Choreoathetosis
    Arm position changes
    Discomfort
Body image
Handedness
    Copy skills: from board/desk
Sensory
    Vestibular
    Tactile
    Auditory
ADLs
    Dressing, feeding, toileting, etc.

ATNR

Asymmetrical tonic neck reflex

STNR

Symmetrical tonic neck reflex

These are stability patterns
necessary for all flow and go
movements.

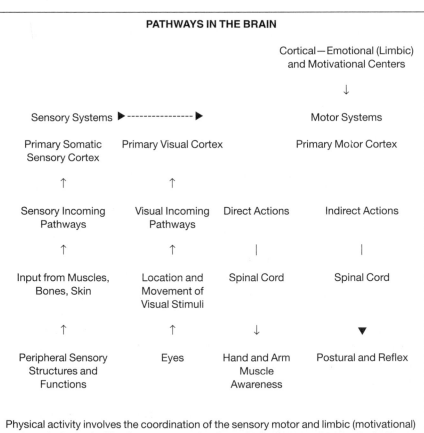

PATHWAYS IN THE BRAIN

Physical activity involves the coordination of the sensory motor and limbic (motivational) systems in the brain. The direct motor pathways make for fast movements, the indirect for slower, more modulated, regulated actions, connected within the nervous system to other associated pathways. Adapted from Kandel, Schwartz, Jessell: Essentials of Neural Science and Behavior, Appleton & Lange, 1995

Pathways in the brain.

Some Frequently Asked Questions

"My kid is the star soccer player. How can he have motor problems?"

The answer: Soccer is a gross motor activity that requires, on the elementary levels, minimal to moderate precision. In addition, because it is a large-motor, constant-movement activity, children with some signs of attention deficits find this "constant go" sport in agreement with the inner moment.

"Why didn't my doctor note this?"

The answer: Physicians are trained to look for systemic and developmental milestone attainment. If the child is well physically and is walking, running, etc. within normal

Put your questions here. If they are not answered, seek out a professional you trust to get those issues addressed.

limits, she may appear "fine." Doctors are not trained to look at the "style" in which a child is accomplishing specific tasks, which is often one of the primary indicators of motor problems.

"Why didn't the preschool teacher alert me?"

The answer: Children attend preschool earlier and earlier in their young lives. Daycare situations are concerned with your child's well-being and happiness. Preschool and kindergarten teachers often see that a child is performing differently from others but may be hesitant to approach the parent for several reasons. Some of the most common reasons are: (1) they are not diagnosticians; (2) they have (probably) not done any formal testing; and (3) often parents become defensive. This is not news parents understand or want to hear. Parents often prefer to believe their child will "outgrow" the problem.

"What is the academic relevance?"

The answer: The academic situation requires that a child be able to fixate, organize, integrate, and feed back specific information in a sequential, logical order. If a child is having difficulty staying in a chair, is poorly organized, cannot cross the midline of his body, and has muscle tone that sends inappropriate signals (e.g., holding the pencil too tightly or too loosely), then performing even the most simple of classroom tasks can become overwhelming. An overwhelmed child becomes a defeated child, and a defeated child fails—even those with superior intelligence.

Occupational therapy helps by giving the child the internal abilities to receive, organize, and utilize required information.

"How is OT compatible and of assistance to classroom situations, tutoring, speech, etc.? Why won't just tutoring help?"

The answer: Tutoring is one-on-one education. That is, more of the same, only individualized. It does not fix neuromuscular problems. Speech, which has its foundation in the neuromotor arena, is a small muscle skill. Often it is important to get the larger muscles to do first what you want the smaller ones to eventually attain.

OT helps in the classroom by giving the child the internal abilities to receive, organize, and utilize required information. OT works on these internal abilities. If the child is not constantly moving, is able to write and read what is written, and can finish work on time, then success in the classroom is enhanced.

Tutoring is important because it reinforces hard-to-grasp concepts and procedures in a private, safe environment.

The *classroom* is important because, in addition to facts, the child learns invaluable social skills.

Speech is important because, in addition to articulation, it teaches receptive and expressive language skills.

OT is important because it teaches the underlying skills and the neuromotor organizational abilities that are at the foundation of all learning.

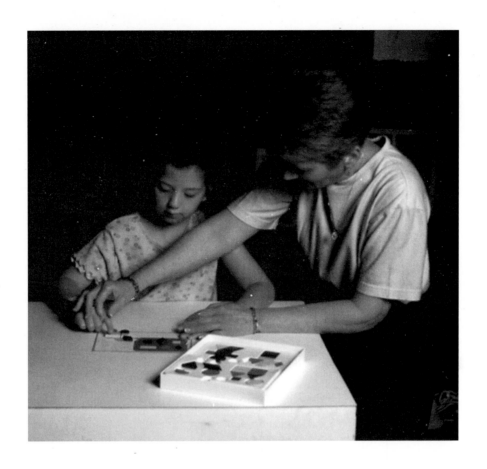

CHAPTER TWO

What is Memory?

Notes

How does your child respond to "old" data and "new" data? What about sequences?

WHAT IS MEMORY?

Memory is the coordination of the senses imprinting on the brain specific sights, sounds, smells, tactile feelings, and emotional feelings.

It is essential for learning.

Three Types of Memory

Immediate

Lasts less than one minute
Contains exact imagery
For retention, information must be transferred to short-term or long-term memory

Short-term Memory

Lasts from a few hours up to a week
Functional brain structures involve the hippocampus, which is the "organizer" of information before it is transferred to the long-term memory.

Long-term Memory

Organization and repetition help store information in the cerebral cortex. Only the basics of the information are stored; many details are obscured.

HOW DO WE REMEMBER?

Touch

Primary sensory input triggers initial memory and excites something called the *somatosensory cortex.*

Sound

Information is stored as it is received in the *primary auditory cortex* within the temporal lobe.

Sight

Encoding of imagery is translated into nerve impulses and sent to the *primary visual cortex.*

Taste and Smell

Receptors in the nose embellish the previously encoded memories to produce enhanced memory "pictures." These are stored in the *olfactory cortex*.

SO..........IF WE HOPE TO REMEMBER WHAT WE ARE TAUGHT, WE MUST STIMULATE THE SENSES TO LEARN.

Possible Behaviors of Students Who Experience Memory Difficulties

Poor organization
Habitual tardiness in turning in assignments
Loss of books, reports, etc
Anxiety
Becoming overwhelmed easily
Freezing up
Sloppiness
Incomplete/insufficient assignments
Working without signs of personal investment
Not following instructions
Overdependence on aid
Becoming distracted easily

These Behaviors Cause the Teachers to Assume that the Student is:

Lazy
Arrogant
Disrespectful
Uncaring
Not working to potential
Inattentive
Excuse-prone
A rule-breaker/rule-tester
Uncooperative
Not trying hard enough

Notes

What is your major concern specific to home?

Specific to school?

Specific to social situations?

Negative halos

What frustrates you when you interact with your child?

What frustrates your child?

What Students with Memory Difficulties are Probably Feeling
Inadequate Awkward Unpopular Defensive Alone Confused Like "everyone" is always staring at them Angry Depressed Emotionally and physically unsafe

If we see it, we recognize it.

If we touch it, we know it.

If we move it, it's ours.

WHAT DOES THE RESEARCH SAY?

Learning is a melding of both art and science. Research in neurobiology confirms that the use of the hands changes the learning process from passive to active, which in turn increases long-term memory, especially that of sequences, and stimulates spontaneous creativity.

Life *is* movement; life *is* dynamic; life *is* a dance for both parents and teachers to learn to dance with these children. So remember that children who experience memory difficulties usually have deficits with immediate and short-term memory and, in addition, these children often have above average to superior long-term memory and, in many cases, above average to superior intelligence.

WOW.

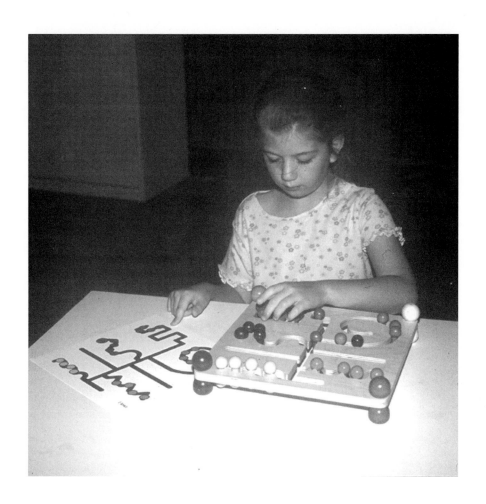

CHAPTER THREE

How We Learn

N o t e s

Emotional Intelligence "is the ability to delay gratification, maintain emotional self-control and be optimistic."

David Hamburg, MD

Psychiatrist, President of the Carnegie Corporation

Learning is really about sensory processing. Emotional components are very important. Peer interactions and social style are strong indicators of possible problems.

Neurologically the emotional center of the brain matures in the following order:

1. Sensory—early childhood

2. Limbic system—puberty

3. Frontal lobes—late adolescence to 18 years of age

The frontal lobes combine the input from the sensory and limbic systems. They are the point of origin of emotional self-control, understanding, and planned responses.

How We Learn

In a report from the National Center for Clinical Infant Programs, a child's readiness for school is directly dependent upon the ability and knowledge of how to learn. How we learn is based on seven traits that impact productive functioning:
1. Confidence—a sense of control
2. Curiosity
3. Intentionality—the wish to be effective and to effect change
4. Self-control
5. Relatedness—to be understood as well as to understand
6. Fluid communication
7. Cooperation with peers and teachers

Optimum performance and learning happen in a state of flow.

Susan N. Schriber Orloff, OTR/L

Emotional Intelligence

Daniel Goleman describes emotional intelligence as involving the following concepts:
1. Knowing one's emotions—self-awareness
2. Managing emotions—handling feelings and building on self-awareness
3. Motivating oneself—using emotions for self-motivation, mastery, creativity, and delaying gratification to reach a goal
4. Recognizing emotions in others—empathy
5. Handling relationships

Data from Goleman D: Emotional intelligence, New York, 1997, Bantam.

Dealing with Emotions

John Mayer, a psychologist from the University of New Hampshire, states that there are three specific ways in which people deal with emotions:
1. Self aware—Aware of moods as they are experienced
2. Engulfed—Swamped by emotions; moods are in charge, not the person
3. Accepting—Resigned to despair or blindly positive; neither have any motivation to change

Data from Goleman D: Emotional intelligence, New York, 1997, Bantam.

Emotions can overwhelm concentration, which is the cognitive ability psychologists often refer to as *working memory*. Working memory occurs in the prefrontal cortex, where feelings and emotions combine.

Anxiety sabotages intellect, inhibits learning, and reduces the quality of judgmental functions.

Good moods enhance flexibility and relaxation, broaden response patterns, and increase problem-solving abilities.

The ability to contain and reframe emotions is called the *master aptitude*.

Children who have learning problems often lack the ability to find the "middle ground." They cannot modulate their physical or emotional selves. An intact modulatory system is at the foundation of being able to store and process information. Modulation gives rise to functional support capacities that give rise to competence with functional end products.

*The word **emotion** is derived from the Latin root meaning "to move." Thus the function of emotions should be to "motivate," to create the possibilities for constructive change, and to provide opportunities for learning new behavioral responses.*

Susan N. Schriber Orloff, OTR/L

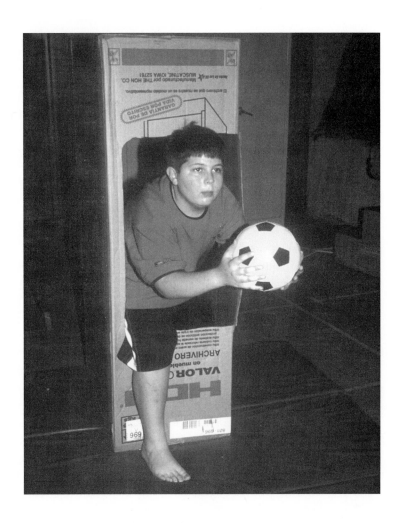

CHAPTER FOUR

Piaget's Theories Simplified

N o t e s

. . . Intelligence is the totality of behavior coordinations that characterize behavior at a certain stage.

Piaget and Knowledge, p. 245

An Overview of Piaget's Developmental Framework

Piaget's theory states that specific age-appropriate learning and behaviors happen in a distinct, predictable progression, all within whatever are the child's general developmental circumstances.

He held that learning and growth are on-going, lifelong processes and that the last stage is perpetually open-ended and evolving. And so, what begins in preadolescence continues in the adult.

The first stage, the *sensory-motor stage,* ending at about age 2, is the most complex, with many substages and marked by reflex, visual awareness, and the graduation from purely random to evident stimuli and from reaction to response.

The second stage, the *preoperational stage,* between ages 2 and 7, is shown by the initiation of the abilities to copy and to accommodate observed behaviors.

The third stage, the *concrete operational stage,* from ages 7 to 11, is the first intellectual growth spurt, with language carrying the principal evidence and allowing the child to evolve communicatively and noncommunicatively.

Communicative speech shares thoughts, feelings, and ideas and includes input from the listener, the other participant in the dialogue.

Noncommunicative speech is a monologue that is often egocentric and repetitive. This aspect of the third stage can be characterized by nonproductive, rambling, unconnected chatter.

The last and longest stage is stage four, the *formal operational stage,* where various intellectual functions spring to greater and greater life. This stage witnesses improvement in the classification of things, the prioritizing of tasks, and sequencing, as well as cinemascopically expanding mental imagery and the development of *equilibrium,* the function that allows a person to put things/events/needs in perspective and keep life on an even keel. *Emotional intelligence,* a term of our time, not Piaget's, fits extraordinarily well here. And he almost certainly would have wished he'd thought of it.

Piaget's Four Stages of Development

Stage One: Sensory-Motor

Birth to 2 years
From random to stimuli-reflexive responses

Stage Two: Preoperational

Age 2 to 7 years
Symbolic play and increased vocabulary

Stage Three: Concrete Operational

Age 7 to 11 years
Sequential ordering, moral judgments, and "fair play"

Stage Four: Formal Operational

Age 11 to adulthood
Emotion, intellect, and equilibrium

Comparison of Llorens, Ayres, Willbarger, and Others with Piaget

Piaget's four stages of development interface easily with the works of Ayres, Llorens, Willbarger, Moore, and others. The theme of four developmental categories, stages, or system processes repeats itself through these many theories and approaches. Ayres's work with sensory integration focuses on the development of the child from a sensory-responsive being to one that produces "functional end products" (i.e., competent, successful cognitive-motor acts in school and at home).

Moore's work with neurodevelopment answers many of the questions of how and why specific responses are often elicited from children exhibiting discrete clusters of cognitive-motor performances.

Text continues on page 32

N o t e s

Understanding the Central Nervous System

1. FRONTAL LOBE
    Planning
    Expressive speech
    Speech
    Movement

2. PARIETAL LOBE
    Touch
    Taste

3. OCCIPITAL LOBE
    Sight

4. TEMPORAL LOBE
    Receptive speech

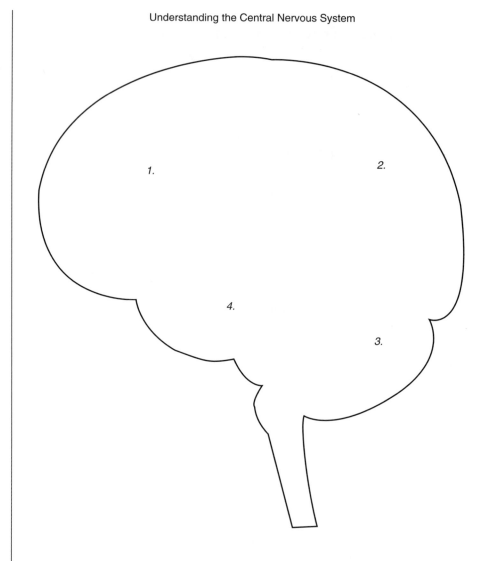

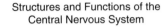

Structures and Functions of the
Central Nervous System

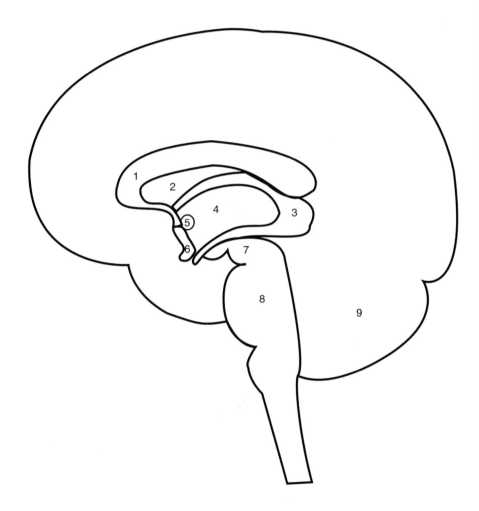

1. CORPUS CALLOSUM
   Allows communication
   between right and left
   sides of brain

2. BASAL GANGLIA
   Controls movement,
   cognition

3. AMYGDALA
   Controls heartbeat,
   emotions

4. THALAMUS
   Relay station to the brain

5. HYPOTHALAMUS
   Controls sex drive/desire,
   temperature, blood
   pressure

6. PITUITARY GLAND
   The "master gland";
   controls hormones/
   growth

7. HIPPOCAMPUS
   Controls long-term
   memory

8. MIDBRAIN
   (Pons, Medulla) Controls
   breathing, circulation,
   digestion, heartbeat

9. CEREBELLUM
   Controls coordination
   of movement

Llorens addresses the areas of sensory input and follows it through the neural pathways to the desired motor output, thus creating a functional feedback system so a specific act may be not only repeated but modified and expanded upon to be utilized in more complex situations.

In each case, these highly respected developmental researchers have demonstrated a consistency in categorizing their theories into four distinct groupings. This consistency cannot be regarded as coincidental when superimposed upon a basic neurological model, which can also be grouped into four areas: (1) central nervous system, (2) peripheral nervous system, (3) sympathetic nervous system, and (4) parasympathetic nervous system.

Utilizing the neurological framework for learning, four sets of developmental skills evolve: (1) sensory-motor, (2) cognitive, (3) psychosocial (intrapersonal), and (4) social (interpersonal) skills. These skills are essential for the creation of, as Ayres would phrase it, "functional end products," or as Llorens would call it, "functional feedback." Whatever it is termed, these are elements necessary for success, not just in school, but in life.

Developing a criterion-referenced assessment that analyzes how a child performs a specific function, in addition to quantitative standardized tests, allows the therapist to utilize the assessment process. The statistical and the inferential data form the foundation for the creation of functionally based goals and treatment.

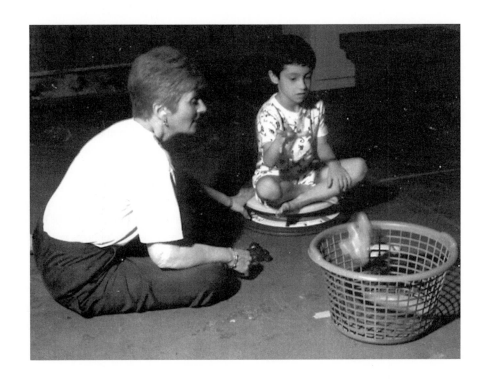

CHAPTER FIVE

Guidelines for Parents

Terms to Know

Visual-motor skills

Ability to visually organize and associate visual stimuli.

Midline development

Development of skills that allow for focal manipulation at the center of the body with peripheral flow from the left to the right as needed for the development of reading and prereading skills.

Peripheral vs focal vision

Normally 80% of the average person's vision is peripheral; 20% is focal. Children with visual-perceptual problems usually have these percentages reversed.

Vestibular disorder

Difficulty in left/right coordination, eye movement, balance, and tactile interpretations. The vestibule is located in the semicircular canals and labyrinths of the ear. Under- or overreactions here can contribute to distorted sensory processing, which in turn can contribute to both behavioral and learning problems.

The How, When, and Why of Occupational Therapy for Parents of School-age Children

Your child might need an occupational therapy (OT) screening if you or the teacher suspects there is a performance gap between him and his peers. Other behaviors in your child that might indicate a need for screening include:

- Becoming frustrated easily

- Rejecting unfamiliar tasks

- Preferring to play alone rather than with friends

- Difficulty transitioning from one task to another

- Poor or slow fine motor skills

- Clumsiness

- Unusual forgetfulness

- Struggling in school

- Allowing social issues to dominate school concerns

- Not wanting to go to school

- Depression

- Poor endurance

Whether we as parents want to admit it or not, our children have us "trained." (And all this time you thought you were bringing them up!) We cue into the moods and needs of our children, often automatically.

An analogy for this might be as follows: Child A lives on Planet Home. It is a nice place and very secure. No matter what Child A does, that he is loved and wanted is never in question. Troublesome behaviors such as incomplete home duties, a messy room, arguments with siblings, forgetfulness, etc., while often followed with a consequence, do not diminish his standing in the family unit.

Child A is also very aware of all the rules, boundaries, and dynamics of Planet Home. And if things get too chaotic, going to a quiet place is usually an option.

This same Child A, who functions so well on Planet Home, often appears to become less competent on Planet School.

New authority figures, different rules, unfamiliar boundaries, new routines, time demands, and strangers (peers and teachers) can make school for children with educational insecurities a very frightening place.

What is OK on Planet Home may not be OK on Planet School. The language may be the same but with different meanings.

Children with learning disabilities often do not transition well from one task/ situation to another, and the average day on Planet School is usually fraught with transitions.

So when the teacher from Planet School observes something that you probably do not see at home, listen carefully. There are most often home behaviors that correlate with those seen in the classroom.

Some Common *Classroom* Signs of Discrete LD

1. Inattentiveness

2. Disorganization

3. Need for repeated instructions

4. Easy frustration

5. Slow work

6. Poor handwriting

7. Social problems (mild to moderate)

8. A child who seems very bright, but just isn't "getting it done"

Some Common *Home* Signs of Discrete LD

1. Problems with dressing and self-care beyond anticipated age of competency

2. Losing personal items

3. Forgetting familiar chores/homework

4. Difficulty with cooperative tasks

5. Difficulty with personal space

6. Oversensitivity with family members and friends

7. Rejecting or excessively fearing slightly familiar or unfamiliar situations

8. Few (new) friends

Functional Checklist

Self-Care

_____ Has problems putting on/taking off coat
_____ Cannot tie shoes
_____ Cannot manipulate buttons, snaps, zippers
_____ Is unkempt
_____ Needs reminders to keep track of belongings
_____ Rejects certain fabrics
_____ Always wears socks; resists bare feet
_____ Habitually wears one or two specific outfits
_____ Other

Motor Skills

_____ Has poor motor learning (new skills)
_____ Has mixed and/or no hand preference
_____ Has poor handwriting
_____ Gets frustrated with fine motor tasks
_____ Has difficulty copying from desk/board
_____ Writing "floats" off the writing line
_____ Has poor gross motor skills (running, jumping, skipping)
_____ Loses place when reading or copying
_____ Has poor grasp (awkward use of pencil/crayon)
_____ Exerts poor writing pressure
_____ Works unusually slowly
_____ Cannot make numbers in a column
_____ Cannot color inside lines as needed
_____ Poorly reproduces shapes/forms/designs
_____ Other

Task Behaviors

_____ Has difficulty staying focused
_____ Is disorganized
_____ Is overly dependent on teacher/parent
_____ Forgets homework
_____ Has poor sequencing skills
_____ Has sloppy desk/notebook
_____ Is easily distracted
_____ Has difficulty initiating tasks
_____ Has difficulty transitioning from one skill/task to another
_____ Needs instructions repeated
_____ Gets confused easily
_____ Is habitually late coming in from activities
_____ Has difficulty skimming page for information
_____ Other

Social Behaviors

_____ Has few friends
_____ Complains that "someone" hit him
_____ Has difficulty with cooperative tasks
_____ Has multiple somatic (physical) complaints
_____ Is hesitant to interact with peers
_____ Has little or no awareness of ambient social cues (e.g., facial expressions)
_____ Has problems lining up with classmates
_____ Has difficulty discerning personal space
_____ Poorly expresses thoughts, ideas, and feelings
_____ Is overly sensitive to corrective remarks (criticism)
_____ Other

Don't jump the gun. If in doubt, get a second opinion from an objective professional.

What have you noticed about your child?

Competencies Needed for School Success

Neurological

Hearing
Balance/gravitational responses
Touch
Sight
Cognition (including attentional issues)

Emotional

Peer interactions
Authority responses
Frustration levels
Task initiation/response patterns
Group skills

Physical

Mobility
Self-care
Hand skills
Strength
Endurance

Intellectual

Performance
Task behaviors (rejection, motivation, curiosity, transitional skills, initiation, organization)
Time concepts (sequencing, getting work done "on time," etc.)
Task production (following directions—verbal, written, demonstrated, repeated, etc.)
Retention (long-term vs short-term memory issues—ADD children)
Task judgments (important to note level of dependence on teacher, peers, self)
Evaluation skills (specific to style and response patterns)

"My child is bright. How can there be learning problems?"

It is not about bright—

In fact, the reason that this child has been able to succeed so far is that she is very bright and has discovered ways to accommodate and facilitate successful outcomes.

Questions Parents Ask

"If my child gets therapy, will the school assume there is something wrong with him and equate this with low intelligence?"

Getting a bright child help helps him from becoming discouraged and defeated. It also breaks the academic mindset that if he only tried harder, he could do it, and that the reason he doesn't is willfulness. A competent therapist will communicate to the classroom teacher just what and why certain techniques are being used so that this can be replicated in the classroom to help ensure increased productivity and success.

"What if I get my child help, and she still has problems? Won't I make things worse if I get accommodations and school issues persist?"

No! Your child is smart enough to know something is not "right." Your child is smart; she already feels "different." With the special service specialist, set realistic expectations for yourself, your child, and the teacher. Ask about what and how long a particular intervention is projected to take. Emphasize to the child that this is not something that is going to be necessarily fast, and that it is not being done *to* her but *with* her full cooperation.

"How do I answer my friends and family when they say I'm overreacting? They tell me I should just let my kid be a kid and that he is bright, and I shouldn't 'stir up stuff'."

The "stuff" is already stirred. Your child receiving help HELPS—period. Old stereotypes and clichés die slow and hard. These individuals are speaking through their own fears and misconceptions. They have not sat in the meetings; they have not read the reports; they have not talked to professionals; and they have not seen the daily turmoil your child is in. Don't listen! You, the parent, have made an informed decision after careful considerations and consultations and in response to your child's expressed (physical, emotional, and/or verbal) discomforts.

"How do I include the educational setting in the therapy process?"

Good communication makes the teacher an integral part of the therapeutic learning process. The chosen method of communication must be agreed upon by the teacher, the parent, and the therapist. Some suggested methods might be email, a "communication book," scheduled phone calls, or meetings. The goals of therapy and those of the school should support each other.

Competence is self-perpetuating and helps . . .

"What should I expect from therapy? When will I notice a change?"

You should expect therapy to be like any new experience for your child. If she adjusts easily to new situations, the start will be more spontaneous than for the child who resists change and/or new situations.

Your child is the KEY member of this team!

N o t e s

Nothing happens without him being consistently present emotionally, intellectually, and physically. Sometimes it will be hard. Sometimes he may feel like nothing is happening.

Acknowledge these very real feelings. He is used to not quite getting "it" right. Emotionally he is prepared to fail, not succeed. An essential part of therapy is to change this "in the rut" thinking.

Your support is essential! Redirect his thinking. Make analogies about something he learned (like riding a bike) that was once hard and is now easy.

Expect stops and starts as therapy progresses. Your child knows she is being brought somewhere to fix something. Although she may want it "fixed," she may resent having to need any type of intervention.

Support the therapy process by explaining why she is going. Don't make it a discussion. This was a decision you made after careful consideration. Don't bargain. This is not negotiable. For therapy to work, the process is initiated in treatment and supported at home. OT "homework" should be taken as seriously as school homework.

Progress depends on commitment.

Changes will be subtle at first. A child who comes to therapy with three shirts on may reduce the need to be covered, indicating a normalization of her tactile system. Another child who is generally a couch potato may want to go out to play; whereas another who is clumsy may demonstrate more agility.

Progress is often met with resistance on the part of the child. This stranger is asking her to give up a way of doing something, however maladaptive, and, on faith, try something new with only the therapist's word that it will be worth the effort to learn and use it.

Traditional learning is hard for your child. She has had problems with it, and now this relative stranger is asking her to learn something unfamiliar in an unfamiliar way in an unfamiliar setting. WOW! This is very threatening to your child. When threatened, people react with rejection, anger, and fear. Your child is no different. That is why your support is vital to the success of therapy.

"Why is my child a wiz on the computer but can't do work in class? Why not just give him a laptop to work with instead of paper and pencil?"
Computers are useful tools after the child has attained adequate in-hand manipulation skills. These skills can only be acquired by using his own hands, and putting his forefinger on a mouse or moving a joystick or an adapted keyboard cannot replace the agility learned through old-fashioned play: jacks, finger painting, hand looms, lacing crafts, etc. Computers reinforce straight-ahead, focal vision-play and not peripheral vision (surrounding side stimuli). A child who does not develop this at a young age may have difficulty picking up on visual cues in the classroom (i.e., blackboard work, following sequences, and visual tracking).

"Why isn't my child having fun in OT, like she did at the beginning? I want my child to be happy!"
There is a difference between happiness and fun. Fun doesn't always add to one's abilities. Happiness is intrinsically related to the attainment of skills and subsequent

feelings of competency, which in turn increase one's emotional security. The path to this security is often hard won. Your job, as parent, is to keep your child motivated through this unfamiliar and challenging process.

Evaluation Elements

Prenotes should include very specific questions. These are often found on the initial intake forms.

Evaluation formats vary. The format below is one that might be used in a variety of settings (school, clinic, or private practice).

Data

Date of evaluation:
Date of birth:
Name:
Parents' names:
Address:
Phone number:
Grade:
Teacher:

Background Information

Psychological tests:
Any special services currently receiving:
Family background:
Illnesses:
Developmental milestones:

Attitude During Tests

Withdrawn:
Attentive:
Hyperactive:
Needed repetition:
Followed directions:
Feared failure:

N o t e s

What is the most important behavioral pattern in your family?

How does (or doesn't) your child express this?

If you could change only one thing, what would it be?

Ask for your "Parents' Bill of Rights" (read it; every state school system has one set up).

If your school system appears to be trying to discourage you from having an evaluation: DON'T GIVE UP. BE PERSISTENT.

Remember that 5 years from now, the only person who will probably still be in your life is your child!

Remember—

This is a snapshot of your child on a particular day, at a particular time. Try to see these specific results in generalities as well as absolutes.

Tests Administered

Standardized:
Formal observations:

Results:

Summary:
Goals:

The following is a sample OT evaluation:

CASE STUDY

Occupational Therapy Evaluation

Name: Sally Jones
Parent(s): Peter and Mary Jones
Address: 1002 Old Road Atlanta,
   GA 32050
Phone: 404-846-0000 (day)
Eval Date: 7-3-00

DOB: 2-1-93
Age: 7.5
Grade: rising 2nd grader
School: Tree-Top Day School
Referred by: L. White, PhD/JFCS

Background Information

Sally is the youngest of three children, and her siblings are much older than she is (ages 17 and 20). By report, all developmental milestones were attained within normal limits, and with the exception of ear infections, health history is not remarkable.

In April 2000, Sally did have a psychological test administered by Dr. L. White at United Family Services. Dr. White referred Sally for an OT evaluation. The results of the psychological testing were not available at the time of this evaluation.

Parents report that she is "reluctant to do worksheets" and "doesn't like to write." In addition to the writing issues, they noted both on the intake form and in the discussion after the evaluation that her task behaviors are a concern. Specifically they note that she has difficulty staying focused, is disorganized and easily distracted, and seems to need instructions repeated more than would be expected.

Behaviors During Testing

Sally initially entered the OT clinic hesitantly, holding her doll "Rita" close to her. After a brief warm-up period to the clinic, she seemed ready to participate in the assessment procedures.

Throughout the testing, she was observed to need both verbal and demonstrated directions repeated and much reinforcement. She appeared to have a significant fear of failure and a hesitancy to engage in unfamiliar tasks. In new situations, there seemed to be an increase in her activity level and a decrease in the quality of her responses. She would often use distracters when presented specific directions. For example, when told to "draw only a person head-to-toe," she added, "I'll first draw a street." She responded well to redirection, but task procedures needed to be repeated using a trisensory (auditory, visual, motor) and structured approach.

Tests Administered

- Wide-range assessment of visual-motor abilities

- Test of visual-perceptual (nonmotor) skills

- Goodenough-Harris drawing test

- ETCH (evaluation of children's handwriting)

- Functional assessment of neuromotor abilities

Results

The *wide-range assessment of visual-motor abilities (WRAVMA)* tests the child in the three spheres of visual-perceptual-motor development. It provides a psychometrically sound assessment of visual-motor, visual-spatial, and fine motor skills. A score of 100 (50%) out of a possible 200 is within the average range (98-103).

Sally's scores were as follows:

Test	Raw Score	Standard Score	Percentile	Age Equiv.
Drawing (visual-motor)	7	72	3	4.10
Matching (visual-spatial)	24	89	23	6.3
Pegboard (fine motor)	29	101	53	7.4*

* On this section, in particular, she often adapted responses and had to restart the task because her changes were not in keeping with the desired action. For example, she wanted to put "order" to the fine motor manipulative test by first selecting only one color and then trying to make a pattern. The instruction was just to fill the pegboard quickly.

This section assesses in-hand manipulation, speed, and accuracy of placement; crossing the body midline; and sustaining a repetitive two-step task pattern and upper extremity stability/mobility patterns. The specific direction was "hold the pegboard with one hand (nondominant) and place the pegs with your other hand, keeping your 'helper' hand on the pegboard so it will not move." Maintenance of these instructions, even after multiple trials, required much repetition and redirection.

It is felt that this is probably due to a visualization and processing interference at this time. At no time did the therapist assess these responses as defiant or willful. Instead it was felt that these were Sally's self-initiated adaptive reactions to try to get the task done as close to "right" as possible.

Her desire to please, her fear of failure, her hesitancy to enter unfamiliar situations, and her success and goal-oriented motivators seem to rule out her responses as "intentional behaviors." Rather, they suggest that her behavior is probably a subcortical response to help her facilitate visual, perceptual, and motor organization.

If this is happening in class, it is probably very frustrating for both Sally and her teachers. She seems to understand the direction, but actually does not, so when she tries to implement it, she changes the procedure, which in turn alters the outcome.

Combined results were as follows: she obtained a composite standard score of 82 and a composite percentage of 12%. Throughout this test she had several behaviors that seemed to negatively impact the results: she would often block the vision of her left eye with the left hand, producing a peering vision response and limiting her ability to respond to a complete visual field. While this was the most observed response, sometimes she would block her right eye with her right hand. This seemed to keep her motor responses one-sided (i.e., she reached for things on her left with her left hand and things on the right with her right hand). Exchange between the right and left hand was not observed, suggesting that activities that require movements across the midline of her body would not be successful at the time of this testing. She frequently twisted and maneuvered in her chair, and she often had to be brought back to the tasks. In addition, she consistently subvocalized what she needed to do, but more as a delay than as an initiator for the item. She was easily discouraged, often saying, "this is hard," needing encouragement to try some items. As previously explained, following specific directions was difficult for her.

The *test of visual-perceptual (nonmotor) skills (TVPS)* tests the seven major visual-perceptual arenas, with the elimination of the motor component. Thus, it is possible to distinguish which is perception and which is motor.

Sally's scores were as follows:

Test	Raw Score	Perceptual Age	Scaled Score	Percentile Rank
Visual discrimination	10	7.5	10	50
Visual memory	9	8.7	11	37
Visual-spatial relationships	14	12.8	14	91
Visual form constancy	9	8.1	11	37
Visual sequential memory	10	7.8	11	50
Visual figure/ground	14	>12.11	18	91
Visual closure	7	7.6	10	16

She received a median perceptual age of 9.2 and an average percentile rank of 58%. The sum of her scaled scores was 73, which gave a perceptual quotient of 103. The perceptual quotient is statistically linked to projected IQ scores, however it is felt that this score is somewhat lower than might be expected due to the range of her performances.

Visual closure, the ability to see half a form on paper and the other half in your head, is crucial for writing, and this was her lowest performance area.

The *Goodenough-Harris drawing test* is a test of fine motor–cognitive/organizational abilities as well as body image. Her raw score was 10, which yielded an age equivalent of 5.2. Although this is slightly higher than her drawing score on the WRAVMA, it is supportive of her issues with visual-motor production. It is important to note that she drew her person with a broken arm. In the drawing, the subject's left arm was in a cast. In addition, when given the instruction to "draw a person," she said, "first I'll draw a street." The therapist had to turn over the paper and have her start on the other side for her to do the task as directed.

Interpretively, using the House-Tree-Person Test criteria, the drawing of an arm that is broken is often suggestive of feeling in some way damaged or limited. Her desire to first "draw a street" may be another indicator of her need to overstabilize within the visual-perceptual realm. Other testing seems to support that she is mostly likely experiencing perceptual place constancy interference.

The TVPS tests only near-point perception. Difficulty seems to come when she has to look at something from a distance or visualize it in her head and then produce it on paper.

The *ETCH* is a standardized test of handwriting performance: evaluating legibility, size, formation, writing line awareness, spacing, and sequencing. A score of 95% is considered fluid writing. She was tested in only the manuscript format.

Her scores were as follows:

Upper-case production	73%
Lower-case production	69.2%
Numbers: 1 to 12	66.6
Near-point copying	60%
Far-point copying	60%
Dictation: numbers	100%[*]
Dictation: letters	33.3%

[*]Although she got all of the numbers in correct order, they were not legible. The 3, 5, and 9 were all reversed, and the 5 and 8 were slanted backwards.

Writing was impacted by omissions, sequencing issues, poor line awareness, and size and spacing concerns. Because the therapist was told in advance that Sally does not like to write, this test was given first to "get it out of the way."

This test supports the previous findings of issues with fine motor ideation to production, referred to as *graphomotor abilities.*

The functional assessment of neuromotor abilities tests how the child approaches, executes, and completes specific developmental tasks. The functional assessment of neuromotor abilities tests the child's functional responses in play/game situations. It factors visual, sensory, motor, and cognitive components of task initiation, organization, and execution.

Her results were as follows:

Vision: tracking was accomplished with minimal head movement but was not easily sustained; convergence was initiated but not completed; holding power was fair, and quick localization needed to be accompanied by auditory stimulation.

Reaching patterns: within normal limits.

Grasp and release: completed with a neutral wrist, both right and left; crossing the midline with both the right and the left, but less frequently with the left; had difficulty following a three-step sequential task.

Bimanual functions: with the exception of cutting skills, all were within normal limits.

Diadochokinesia (rapid forearm rotations): irregular and labored in all modes.

Isolated finger control: within normal limits.

Range of motion: within normal limits.

Hand strength: within normal limits.

Flexor/extensor control: can assume positions, but had difficulty maintaining both prone and supine positions for more than 5 seconds.

Muscle tone: completed with overstabilization.

Equilibrium: tested in the static mode; completed with fast displacement (again supporting the earlier findings of overstabilization, suggesting diminished tone).

Upper extremity stability/weight shift: unstable; difficulty assuming and/or maintaining the weight on arms/hands position.

Primitive motor reflexes: (these should have been resolved by 18 months of age); all were present.

Functional movement patterns: difficulty ascending and descending stairs, running, hopping, and skipping.

Standing balance: impaired with both eyes open and closed.

Schilder's arm extension: completed with extreme rigidity; elbows in hyperextension with both trunk rotation and head rotation.

Body image: intact.

Crossing the midline: more on the right than on the left, but generally stayed one-sided; did not cross the midline of her body during motor tasks.

Dominance: established on the right; when writing she habitually did not hold the paper with her left; held her head instead; tended to be perfectionistic; writing was accomplished with an intense four-finger thumb-wrap grasp.

Copy skills: appeared to lose her place easily, more so with far-point copying than with near-point.

Work pace: had to be constantly monitored; seemed to "freeze" when unsure of a response; "best guessing" was very hard for her.

Sensory responses: stereognosis (identification of familiar object with vision occluded by touch only) within normal limits; position sense grossly intact; proprioception (muscle/bone/joint awareness) impaired as was localization of tactile stimuli; vestibular (nystagmus) responses; depressed; there was no nystagmus after first and second rotations.

Dressing skills: dependent (by report).

Summary

Sally initially presented as a very shy child who responds well to structure and support. She appeared to be trying her best throughout the testing situation, but she seemed to become easily intimidated when situations were unfamiliar.

Following directions, both verbal and demonstrated, required sample "practices"and additional repetitions. She seemed to distract herself from the specific tasks, changing them (in an engaging manner) so that she was then following her own agendas. When structured into a specific pattern, she exhibited fatigue response.

Sally does not appear to have visual constancy, which means that things are constantly shifting within her visual field. It is felt that this is contributing to many of her observed task behaviors. If things in her world are constantly shifting, then to find her "place," she seems to have adopted a rigid and self-directed pattern. "If I can't follow the exact direction, then I will come as close to it as I can" seems to be her current task style.

This is probably very frustrating for both Sally and her teachers. Asking her to do specific tasks that always appear to "almost" get done probably produces dissatisfaction on the part of the teacher and a feeling of defeat for Sally.

In the sensory realm, Sally also exhibited problems with touch localization, balance, and coordination. There appears to be a discontinuity between her accessing a visual "steady state" and the planning of required motor responses, both gross and fine.

A program of OT intervention is suggested to help remediate these concerns.

As therapy will begin this summer, suggestions for the classroom teacher will be made closer to the start of school. In addition, it is suggested that at the start of the school year the direct therapist visit the school to observe the classroom and meet with both the parents and the teachers to discuss this evaluation and subsequent suggestions.

Goals

1. Normalize tone

2. Increase ability to follow directions, including sequencing skills

3. Increase visual-perceptual skills

4. Increase fine and gross motor planning

5. Increase cutting skills

6. Increase organizational and sequencing abilities, building to a three-step nonrepetitive pattern

7. Increase writing abilities, starting with the "Calaerobics" worksheets, and then moving into the cursive Handwriting Without Tears program

It may be helpful to consider a speech therapy evaluation to assess auditory processing abilities.

Children need to move! Limit computer time!

It has been a pleasure to evaluate Sally. It is suggested that this report be shared with the referring psychologist, teachers, pediatrician, and other related health professionals.

Susan N. Schriber Orloff, OTR/L

Toys that Facilitate Required School Competencies

Toys that have multiple sensory components to which children are required to respond are best. Many of the toys in therapy catalogues can be found as less expensive versions in places like Target, Wal-Mart, and Toys R' Us, so don't rush to order. Instead use the pictures in the catalogues to find similar toys. They do not have to be exact duplicates to be good.

There are no toys that just do one thing. There are toys that do one thing more than another. However, on the main, common parental/therapeutic/academic sense prevails best.

Neurological competency can be stimulated by toys that encourage and or require touch, movement, sound responsiveness, and balance with expanding attentional demands and visual tracking.

People do not automatically learn to run. We fall down, we get up, and we try again. Children must be provided with the opportunity to develop their own personal sensory systems. Games teach children in a subliminal way how to mature. Some oldies but goodies are "Blind Man's Buff," "Marco Polo," monkey bars, climbing equipment, tug of war games, etc.

These competencies evolve over time with repeated and varied experiences.

Emotional learning is paramount to all the other learning that we do, and it is ongoing throughout life.

We must teach our children to be social. We exist in groups. Games that they can play against themselves to get their "personal best" as well as those they play with one or two others are excellent. Look for short-term games for the younger children. Remember that a 4-year-old child has an attention span of about 4 minutes, so keep it novel and keep it short.

Some suggested toys that meet the above criteria are:

Bop It

Simon

Bumble Ball

Wiggly Giggly Ball

Rapper Snappers

Tactile Dominoes

Koosh Balls

Tactile balls

Whistle straws

Think & Go toys (farm, city, etc.)

Balance beams (you can make one with a 2×4 from the lumber/hardware store)

Old appliance boxes lined with rug samples make great "hideaways"

Zip lines

Rocking/Sliding/Turning toys, such as Dizzy Disc

Yarn blowpipes

Ring-toss

Jump rope

Jacks

Board games
    Chutes and Ladders
    Checkers

Scrabble Jr.
Clue

Other games
    Connect Four
    Battleship

Easels and paints

Tetherball

Rebounder

This is only a starter list and should not be considered a complete mandate for acceptable toys.

Resources for Toys and Equipment

Achievement Products for Children (1-800-373-4699)
Developmental toys made for numerous children to use over time; good for therapy clinics

Back to Basics Toys (1-800-356-5360)
Good old-fashioned kid-powered toys

Cognitive Therapeutics Catalog (1-800-444-9482)
Interactive (anger, family relationships, academics, etc.) board games for children ages 8 to 16

Constructive Playthings (1-800-448-7830)
Manipulative toys, problem-solving toys, etc.

Fun Express (1-800-875-8494)
Similar to Oriental Trading Company, but mainly bulk orders

Hammacher Schlemmer (1-800-892-1063)
Various hard-to-find adaptable items.

Kaplan: Concepts for Exceptional Children (1-800-334-2014)
Good source for large foam ramps, seating options, puzzles that are disability-inclusive

Kinetic Kids (1-800-622-0638)
Variety of toys and tools to teach sensory and life skills

Lakeshore Learning Materials (1-800-421-5354)
Good resource for parents, teachers, and therapists; wide range of toys and prices

Lekotek Toy Resource Helpline (1-800-366-PLAY)
Also have "lending toy libraries"

Lily's Kids (1-800-545-5426)
Wide variety of toys that can be used in multiple ways; toys for gross to fine motor skills; puppet theater, etc.

Oriental Trading Company (1-800-228-2269 or 1-800-875-8480)
Bulk toys for clinics, parties, etc.

OT Ideas, Inc. (1-973-895-3622)
OT supplies for teaching fine motor skills

Play with a Purpose (1-407-872-3838)
Focus on gross-motor development, interactive toys

Pocket Full of Therapy (1-800-PFOT-124)
Multiple gadgets and games for facilitating classroom activities

pro.ed (1-800-897-3202)
Products for special education, rehabilitation, gifted children, and children with developmental disabilities

Professional Development Programs (1-651-439-8865)
Sensory processing, postural control, skill development toys

S & S Opportunities (1-800-243-9232)
Adapted play toys, mats, exercise equipment, and inflatables

Sears Christmas Wishbook
An oldie but goodie

Sportime Abilitations (1-800-850-8602)
Mainly gross motor games and toys

Sunburst Technology (1-800-321-7511)
Graded computer games that teach typing and other needed skills

Therapy Shoppe (1-800-261-5590)
A variety of economically priced fine motor and creative toys; inexpensive and unusual therapy

Therapy Skill Builders (1-800-211-8378)
Videos and skill-specific toys; good evaluation selections

Troll Learn and Play (1-800-247-6106)
Manipulative and make-believe toys, arts and crafts, some toys for gross-motor
  skills

Development programs for schools, organizations, groups, etc.

Advanced Rehabilitation Services, Inc. (1-770-973-3466)
Chris Bosonoto Doane, President
413 Indian Hills Trail
Marietta, GA 30068

Provides services for professionals with continuing education credits for occupational therapists, physical therapists, speech therapists, and teachers.

INDIVIDUAL EDUCATION PLAN
What is an Individual Education Plan?

Individual education plan (IEP) is a term used in all public schools. In private schools it can be called a variety of names: student education plan (SEP), committee of education concerns (CEC), recommended plan, etc. No matter what it is called, it is a binding document that requires teachers to make specific accommodations and modifications to compensate for a child's identified issues or deficits and to facilitate learning. It should include measurable goals and methods for accomplishing specific skills. It should be time-specific and have a designated review period. It needs to be signed by both parents and teachers. If there is disagreement, a process for resolution and mediation should be in place and can be requested by either party.

Parents' rights are discussed later. It is suggested that county and/or state requirements be reviewed prior to any meeting. A copy of these policies can be obtained at the public school or the state's Department of Education.

Questions to Ask at an IEP Meeting

Outline the problem

What are the child's strengths and weaknesses, and how are they impacting the functional outcomes in the classroom?

Goal statements

Are the goals measurable? Will the child be able to accomplish the required tasks in a specific amount of time with an anticipated degree of accuracy?

Analysis of the problem

Have the team members generated and tested hypotheses related to the stated problems in an attempt to determine why the problem is occurring?

Intervention design

Based on the hypotheses of why these problems are occurring, what strategies are going to be used, and do they follow a developmental sequence?

Evaluation and selection of interventions

What are the priorities? Who will be implementing what?

Implementation

Selected interventions are monitored for effectiveness. Who monitors what?

Evaluation of outcome

Final step: compare the child's current abilities with those at the onset of the intervention, measure what progress has and has not been made, and state why. Also determine what needs to be done next.......

IEP "Game Rules"

- Don't be afraid to be an advocate for your child.

- Don't be intimidated. Public schools generally have overworked agendas. That is not your problem; it is theirs. What is expedient for them may be very wrong for your child.

Prioritize your objectives. Be ready to compromise.

- Know the law(s), and make your requests within the law. Schools have to do what is written.

- Come into the meeting with your facts in order.

- If you invite specialists, make sure the school is informed ahead of time, or the person may not be allowed into the meeting.

- You don't have to sign anything at the meeting. Get a second opinion; take time to think. If nothing happens of use or acceptability, you have the right to postpone the meeting.

- You have the right to object and/or ask for clarification.

- Don't be afraid of being labeled a "troublesome parent." Be afraid of *not* being labeled it, sooner or later. The child needing your help had best have a meddlesome, adamant, inexorable parent. In fact, if you don't eventually find yourself with one of these labels, you are either too "agreeable" or are extraordinarily lucky in your dealings with public school bureaucracy.

- You have the right to request specific testing (standardized, criterion-referenced, and functional) and for it to be done within the designated time limits of the law of the state or county.

- You have the right to have testing done again for validity, but read evaluations as a guide, not an indictment. It can help to keep goals realistic and minimize frustration for all.

- You have the right to have requests and responses documented. You do not have to just take school representatives at their word. You should get a copy of everything written about your child; verbal agreements are nonexistent.

- You have the right to ask why something is being recommended. You should also ask when, how, and by whom.

- Seek outside help if needed. Special education services are often put into the curriculum as related support services. This means that your child will only get help if he meets certain criteria. The average child with a learning disability is too "smart" for services and too "problematic" for systems that teach to the mean majority.

- Teach your child to stand his ground. If something doesn't sound right to him, he DOES NOT have to accept it without checking with you. He can always call you to ask you if something sounds or feels right.

- But if the IEP team writes it, they must do it. No alterations, changes, or modifications can be made by them without your prior knowledge and approval.

- You have the right to question specific grades.

- You have the right to a syllabus of each subject.

- You have the right to know what your child will be graded on and how each item will be weighted.

- You have the right to a conference at any time.

- You have the right to limit the scope of the conference to a specific concern.

- You have the right to end a conference if it is not in keeping with the intent of the called meeting.

- Do not keep the meeting going on forever. Teachers are not being paid by the hour, but treat them as if you are the one paying. They have families and lives outside of school, and their time should be respected. If more time is needed for resolution or closure, ask for a continuation.

- You have the right to expect your concerns to be taken seriously and respectfully by the rest of the IEP team, and you should reciprocate.

- You have the right to expect the school to teach both to your child's present performance level and to his assumed potential (by testing and observation.)

- You should not "bulldozer" the meeting. Make sure the right to speak and be heard is extended to both you and the rest of the IEP team.

- Come into the meetings prepared to compromise, but know your "bottom line."

- Do not allow a school official to be punitive. You can take your concerns to his or her supervisor.

N o t e s

- Your child should not be singled out because he is receiving accommodations.

- Your child should NEVER be threatened, be made fun of, or isolated because of modifications.

- Find an ally on the faculty and get advice from that person. "Inside information" can be invaluable.

- Don't be afraid to be human. This is your child. He is hurting, and you are hurting for him. Your objective is to get the kind of help that will ultimately get your child to the point of independence—not just in school but in life. You are not out to change the system, just to use it in the best way possible for the benefit of all. For if the child succeeds, the school does too.

- Talk about feelings. School learning is about social as well as academic growth.

We are who we are forever. Our responses are what we can change. Teachers and therapists cannot cure a learning disability.

- Be motivated by true concern, not control. This is not about power but about *empowerment* for your child and the teacher.

- Reasonable progress commensurate with your child's innate abilities is the only real goal, but goals that are written on the IEP should be time-specific and measurable.

- Remember you are an expert too. Who else at that table really loves your child? So make sure that you are a full participant of the team. You don't have to "take it or leave it."

- If at all possible, parents, guardians, or significant others should present themselves as a united front. When the rest of the IEP team sees you united, they will often stand behind you more readily.

- If you would call for apologies, then also provide them if called for.

- Say thank you.

" . . . A copy of the report sent to private school is requested under the Freedom of Information Act. No documents written on behalf of my child can be withheld from me, his legal guardian . . . "

- Give praise to the school officials and the teachers, not just complaints.

- All of us march to our own beat; make sure your child knows that his beat is not wrong or odd, just unique. And remind him that what is at one time unique often becomes the standard later. Each star has its place in heaven, some just have to move around a bit to find the right spot. Read *Leo the Late Bloomer* together often and talk about it.

How to Have a Successful IEP Meeting

1. Have the right mindset.

This meeting is your meeting. The primary persons are you and your child, not the teachers. You are the expert on your child.

2. Talk from the heart.

This is not about wanting to control the school or the committee. This is about your *fears* and your *dreams* for your child. This is about what your child *fears*, and what he *dreams*.

Go in with a prepared list of your concerns. It is easy to get intimidated by the number of experts around the table. Again, you are the expert on your child.

Below are samples of statements that may correspond to your situation:

Fears:

- The classes my child is in now will limit her choices when she is older.

- The situation he is now in makes him feel like a loser.

- The peer group with whom she is placed has a negative influence.

- I have noticed the following changes in his behavior. (List them)

- She has all but given up. How can I help her want to learn?

- He is feeling rejected by both teachers and peers.

- I am afraid of these feelings of alienation.

- She seems depressed.

- His eating habits have changed. (Fear of eating disorders)

"Uh oh, another thing for me to deal with!"

If you could get help with only a few functional concerns, what would they be?

- Her potential is not being addressed.

- His limitations are not being accommodated properly.

- She is spinning her wheels. I do not see any learning or growth.

Dreams:

- I want him to have friends.

- I want her to feel like she belongs at the school, like she has a niche.

- I want him to feel like someone cares.

- I want her to feel that despite her current level of functioning, someone has faith that she can make and reach her goals.

- I want him to feel he can exceed, succeed, and thrive.

- I want her to feel connected to the learning process, the teachers, and the school.

- I want him to feel that there is something special about him that is positive and unique.

- I want her to feel liked.

- I want him to be able to make the right choices in peer situations.

- I want her to know how to discriminate between potentially positive and negative situations.

- I want him to feel that he can try something slightly beyond his reach and that there are teachers here to help him.

- And when this "growing up" is over, I want her to be an independent, content, goal-directed, successful adult.

3. **Set the IEP goals based on these dreams and fears.**

4. **Make the goals specific.**

5. **The goals should be measurable. (He will do _____ by [date/time].)**

6. Now ask the rest of the IEP team how they can help you and your child reach these goals.

7. A communication system should be established for you to reach a key person of the team if you have questions and/or concerns.

8. Everything should be in writing; accept no oral promises.

9. Do not sign anything you are unsure of. You have the right to clarification.

10. You have the right to convene a meeting or adjourn one *for any reason.*

11. You have the right to bring other experts into the meeting as long as the school is notified in advance.

12. Older children may want to be present. This often works against you, as the team may feel they have to "talk tough," and the meeting can inadvertently become a power struggle. Let your child come in briefly, if he or she insists, either at the end or beginning of the meeting.

Final Note

These people are being p*aid;* they are not your friends; they are not permanent in your life; you do not have to please them. But be polite. Keep focused on your goals. Get them, if at all possible, on your "dream team." They are in the "successful kid business," so let them show you what they've got! Let them help you make your dreams, and those of your child, come true.

End-of-year IEP Questions to Ask

1. What was the original status, and how was that determined?

2. Initiating course work: *How* did it address initial strengths and weaknesses? *What* adaptive techniques were used that were different from traditional teaching/learning techniques?

3. How was he after 6 weeks? After 3 months? After 6 months? Now?

4. What were the specific weaknesses that were initially observed (not included in recent IEP)?

If you have your child in private school, you are still entitled to all of this information. You can request testing and services.

5. *How* and *when* were they resolved?

6. What methods did you use? (Be specific)

7. What is the current status?

   Academic (how does this correspond to standardized state requirements for each grade level?)

   Reading
   Math
   Language arts
   Science

   Intellectual

   Performance
   Task behaviors
   Time concepts (sequencing, getting work done on time)
   Task productions (following [repeated] verbal, written, and demonstrated directions)
   Task judgments (independent or relies on teacher or friends? secure or insecure?)
   Retention (long-term vs short-term)
   Organization
   Comprehension
       Auditory
       Reading
       Visual
       Directional
   Evaluation skills (how he accepts critical assessments, self-evaluations, etc.)

   Physical

   Mobility (getting from one needed place to another [on time])
   Self-care
   Hand skills
   Strength
   Endurance

   Emotional

   Response to authority figures
   Frustration levels (if there is a problem here, please be specific and list the primary and secondary concerns and how they are manifested during the school day in academics, lunch room, art, music, physical education, etc.)

Task response behaviors: avoidance; passivism; fearfulness; requiring (circle one):
normal   somewhat more than average   excessive help from teacher

How does he ask for it?

Does he notice the needs of peers?

Can he wait his turn?

Is he easily distracted? Select one: *noise   visual interference   both*

Sensitivities? How are they addressed in the classroom? When do they regularly appear? How fast are they resolved? When are they appropriate? When are they not?

How did you reach these determinations? What standardized and criterion-referenced standard observational forms/tests did you use? How did you select them and why?

Plans? For what? How will they be implemented?

HOMEWORK

Homework . . . Parents hate it. Kids hate it. What to do?

Homework is the *number one* thing that parents and children fight about. The scenario, with some variation, usually goes something like this:

Parent: *How was your day at school?*
Child: *OK*
Parent: *What did you do?*
Child: *Not much*
Parent: *Do you have homework?*
Child: *Did it in school.* or *Don't have any.*

To be realistic, some homework can be done in school, especially if there are study periods. However most of it does need to be done at home, hence the term *homework.*

Lately there has been a lot of controversy over what the value of homework is, how much is too much, and how much is not enough. However until some major policy is formulated, the homework issue looms large within the family dynamic.

Teachers pass out notes to be taken home. Agendas are filled out with assignments. Permission slips are often stuffed into a bookbag, never to be seen again.

Transportation, location (your child's private school or his home-based facility), and timing will need to be negotiated. Never be afraid to ask.

In all of this there is one abiding truth: in order to do homework, the bookbag must be opened.

This is crucial, and even more so for the child with learning issues. She spends a lot of her day trying to avoid being called on, picked on, and singled out. She is a master at being nearly invisible.

Learning for the child with a learning disability is often fraught with problems, and the "monsters" inside that bookbag are just tangible reminders of his difficulties.

Although the suggestions listed here work for all children, they are particularly helpful for children with learning disabilities.

"Homework Survival Kit"

The basic concept is to get the bookbag opened and the contents reviewed *daily*. It is of paramount importance to say that an established firm routine is essential.

Taking into consideration the many variances of children and their families, the following basic framework is suggested:

I call it the "Homework Survival Kit." You will need to select a place that is not in the child's room—a "portable office." When isolated, the learning-disabled child often drifts into random thoughts or becomes frozen, unable to start the assignments. Choose a place such as the dining room, or put a card table up close to but separate from the family action (kitchen, den, etc.). Let the child know she can ask questions and call for help, and that you will be checking in on her as needed.

Parents will need to supply two moderately sized boxes with lids and a Tupperware-type container for the pantry.

Preferably with the child, select two different patterns of contact paper. With the child's participation, cover each box inside and out, including the top, with contact paper. This will become the child's *Supply Box,* and will include all supplies generally needed for homework. The other box is for all the contents in the bookbag, and will become the *Homework Box.* The Tupperware-type box will serve as the Snack Box, and will be filled with snack foods and kept in the pantry.

A suggested routine might be as follows:

1. Get home with bookbag and empty it into the Homework Box.

2. Put Supply Box on selected table/area.

3. Set up the portable office space.

4. Put the bookbag on the floor near the chair where the child will be working.

5. Have a snack/relax/play (i.e., decompress from the school day).

6. Put the Snack Box on the homework table.

7. Put notes that need to be signed and returned in a Parent Box (a tray in which all notes that need signatures are placed).

8. Refer to student agenda or other lists to determine the homework assignments.

9. Put them in an order such as spelling first, math second, etc. in the Homework Box.

10. Complete one assignment at a time.

11. As they are completed, return the assignment and the corresponding book to the bookbag.

12. When the Homework Box is empty, put all the supplies back into the Supply Box.

13. Return the Snack Box back to pantry.

14. Put the Homework Box and the Supply Box away (preferably in a closet, out of sight).

Supply Box contents:

- Scotch tape

- Stapler

- Electric pencil sharpener

- Paper: plain, lined, and graph

- Rulers: one 6″ and one 12″

- Children's dictionary

- Electronic speller

- Tag board for table (to make a smooth writing surface)

- Glue sticks

- Scissors

- Pencils

- Pens

- Colored pencils

- Crayons

- Markers

- Hole punch and hole reinforcements

- Folders

- Large (5″×8″) envelopes

- Small expandable file

- Calculator

- Small desk lamp

- Extension cord

Snack Box contents:

- Something salty (chips, pretzels, etc.)

- Something sweet (candy, dried fruit, etc.)

- Something chewy (gum, Twizzlers, etc.)

- Something to drink (juice, water, etc.)

- Napkins

- Paper plates

- Cups

Additional necessities:

- Comfortable chair (at right height for table)

- Knowledge of your student: does he work best isolated or near others? Let him choose the most productive spot (not in front of the television).

Allow for a few limited breaks to sustain motivation. Your child will, over time, establish her own work rhythm.

She can get ready in stages so by the time she sits down, the organization stage has given her a system for ferreting out not just what needs to get done, but how to do it as well.

How to Increase the Effectiveness of the Homework Survival Kit

ESSENTIAL PERFORMANCE COMPONENTS

1. Meaning

Besides just getting it done, can your child put understanding both the *what* and *why* of the assignment? Resistance is usually not about power but about *fear* (a fear often not yet acknowledged by the child). The child is dodging *discomfort*, not *work*.

2. Function

What will it help your child do better? (This can be unrelated to the task, such as feeling comfortable around peers in her class or when she gets an assignment back.)

3. Form

Is your child proud of the results?

Remember school is her *job*, her *workplace*. The same elements that are necessary for you to feel good at work are needed for her to feel good at school.

Getting started

Before your student starts to work:

- Help her get organized (put out books, assignments, etc.)

- Be with her as she sets up her "office"

- Be within easy reach if she needs to ask a question once she is working

- Help her visualize the results, not just getting it done

- Let her know you are available for help

- Sit with her for a short time at the start of the homework session

As she is working:

- Go over instructions for assignments if needed

- Be supportive, but do not do the work for her!

- Have her bring you each piece as it is done

- Encourage self-evaluation skills

- Help her put homework in her bookbag for the next day

- Acknowledge how hard this is for her; praise her efforts

- Help her keep track of time and pace her work

Finishing up

When tasks are completed:

- Help her put away her Homework Survival Kit.

- Allow for some downtime.

- Reading to her, talking with her, and "alone" time can be very empowering for a child who is demonstrating homework aversion.

- Remember as her confidence increases, the need for your involvement will decrease, which translates into more personal free time for you.

FINAL NOTES

Do not "rescue" your child; give her the resources to be able to continually design and redesign herself. For life is all about change—constant, inevitable, continual.

Life situations will be sometimes positive and sometimes negative. A successful person is able to learn and grow from both experiences.

Life's path will be both smooth and rough. The ability to be able to know how and when to right oneself is part of life's learning process, and it is only learned individually. It is essential for emotional health.

It is only with a feeling of well-being that permanent, positive learning occurs.

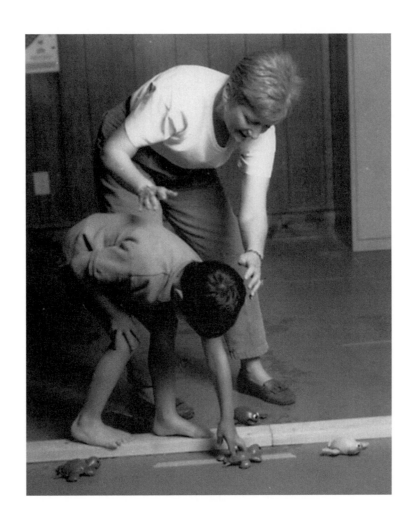

CHAPTER SIX

Guidelines for Teachers

Developmental Markers for Preschool Children

Age	Gross Motor	Fine Motor	Social
1 year	Gets up fast unassisted	Throws things on floor often	Five-to ten-word vocabulary
	Walks unassisted	Builds tower of two cubes	Jargon
	Creeps up stairs	Holds two cubes in one hand	Names a few pictures
	Squats to play	Likes putting things in/out	Understands simple verbal commands
	Hurls ball	Scribbles spontaneously	Two-word phrases
		Uses spoon in feeding	Good movement of tongue, lips, and palate
		Turns two to three pages at once	
		Takes off shoes and socks	
2 years	Walks/runs fairly well	Turns door knob	Refers to self by name
	Walls up/down stairs two feet at a time	Washes and dries hands	Simple sentences and phrases
	Kicks large ball	Builds tower of six to seven cubes	No jargon
	Picks up objects from floor	Imitates making cube train	Begins to match objects or pictures
	Heel-to-toe gait	Puts on shoes, socks, pants	Plays meaningfully with dolls and toys
	Toilet trained/dry at night if taken to toilet	Imitates drawing vertical line and crude circle	Begins to use pronouns
	Walks on tip toes in play	Overhand grasp	Begins to verbalize about immediate experiences
	Jumps with both feet	Snips with scissors	Chooses meals
		Strings beads	
		Turns pages one-by-one	
		Unscrews toy nut and bolt	
		Recognizes primary colors	
3 years	Walks up stairs with alternating feet	Holds pencil in hand instead of fist	Answers comprehensive questions
	Walks down stairs two feet at a time	Removes shoes and pants	Knows gender
	Jumps from bottom step with both feet	Unbuttons, unlaces, unzips	Uses plurals
	Stands on one foot/balances for a moment	Feeds self with little spilling	Identifies use of things in pictures
		Puts three shapes in formboard	Names ten objects in picture and use

	Gross Motor	Fine Motor/Adaptive	Language/Social
	Rides tricycle using pedals	Builds tower of ten cubes	Repeats three numbers
	Catches ball with arms extended	Imitates drawing crude circle	Recognizes accomplishments
		Draws crude man on request	Has attention span of 2 to 4 minutes
		Matches primary colors	
4 years	Throws ball overhand (dominance begins to be evident)	Eats independently	Follows two-step direction
	Stands on one foot for 2 seconds	Dresses and undresses	Names primary colors
	Tries to hop	Laces shoes	Speaks in complete sentences
	Jumps on toes	Buttons	Speech is understandable
		Copies cross and circle	Is less anxious to please
		Washes hands and face	
5 years	Hops on one foot; skips	Ties shoes	Follows three-step request
	Walks upstairs with alternating feet/marches	Copies square	Correctly uses parts of speech
	Stands on each foot with eyes open for 5 to 10 seconds	Cuts on straight line	Counts ten items
	Stands on each foot with eyes closed for 10 seconds	Draws recognizable man	Can group four out of ten items
		Upon request, tries to stay between lines when coloring	Gives name, age, and address
		Nests boxes correctly	Has 5-minute attention span
		Copies triangle (6 yrs)	Likes to please
		Copies diamond (7 yrs)	
		Can walk backward heel-to-toe	

Some of the common "glass half empty" views . . . 👉

and some of the "glass half full" views . . . 👉

Possible Teacher Reactions to a Child with Special Needs:

- Forget about her

- Phone her parents

- Complain

- Punish her

- Give her just the minimum because "she'll never get it anyway"

- Talk to her and find out how work is being done

- Have her keep a work log for 2 to 3 days

- Help her brainstorm strategies for improved efficiency

- Use a behavior checklist/interest inventory to promote discovery of work/study styles

- Suggest testing

- Be supportive

Age-based Activities for School Success

School Competencies: *Neurological*

- Hearing
- Balance
- Gravitational responses

- Tactile
- Visual
- Cognitive (including of attentional issues)

Suggested Activities:
Localization of various sounds in movement games • Treasure hunts • Climb and slide under/over tables chairs • Looking at mystery pictures while leaning over a table upsidedown • Arranging a pattern while hanging upsidedown • Matching/sorting games • Finishing pictures and/or patterns • Choosing a cause or an effect of a situation (e.g., if the drinking glass is left near edge of the table, what are the possible results? [Results can be acted out or drawn] • Utilizing unfamiliar ways (e.g., balance beams in various configurations)

AGE 3	AGE 4	AGE 5
Keep it simple	Add some independent decision-making	Require some guided independent decision-making
Give no more than two to three repetitive directions so that a pattern can be established and repeated	Example of group instructions: First pair of steps repeated, second pair of steps repeated, then first pair repeated again	Make some directions nonrepetitive and sequential
Walk them through the pattern at least two times, and then offer assistance as needed	Keep tasks within specific time limits	Include sorting tasks that require cross-referencing (e.g., items that are rough in texture and used in the kitchen)
Expect some hesitations	Ask students to do some things with their eyes closed	Play "telephone" motor games that require students to remember and add to the list of things to do
Expect some impulsive responses; expect some parallel play	Ask students to change postures	
Provide clear structure	Change the way a familiar object is used, such as a chair, a step stool, etc.; make tunnels and bridges to cross over	Ask students to recall movements with eyes closed
Keep it short; multiple short-term tasks are more readily responded to than one longer task	"Buddy" the kids with partners	Upgrade all previous activities

School Competencies: *Emotional*

- Peer interactions
- Authority responses
- Frustration levels

- Task initiation/response patterns
- Group skills

Suggested Activities:
Leadership activities • Role playing and dramatizations (e.g., use empathy; pretend you are old, blind) • Follow the leader with alternate leaders • Games that require the use of their full name and /or age • Memory recall games • Integrating new words for language enrichment • Time limitations and awareness • Ordinal awareness • Prepositional understandings with directions • Observational skills • Personal space games (e.g., use hula hoops, etc.)

AGE 3	AGE 4	AGE 5
Remember that attention span is 2 to 4 minutes	Expect awareness of left and right with visual assists	Remember that attention span is 5 minutes or more
Ask one-part questions; seek immediate answers	Play games in which two parts make a whole	Do shared activities
Have students find picture-specific items for different categories (e.g., things we eat, things we wear, things that are blue, concrete things found in a bathroom, den, etc.)	Have students make choices (e.g., "You are going on a trip and you want to take all these things [show students several items], but you only have room for three. Which will you choose and why?")	Do sequential tasks that require waiting for each student's turn to come around again
		Play trust activities with parachutes, blankets, etc.
Have students work in groups; each person should have a specific task	Play junkbox activities (e.g., "What would you use this thing for?"; set up "in need" situations)	Do unfamiliar tasks with no clear solutions; have the group decide how something should be done
Play classroom "Monopoly" on the floor; have students move about and buy and/or control certain blocks; talk about feelings	Have students take turns being blindfolded, walk around with a friend, and let the friend describe something without naming it while trying to guess the object	Play verbal and motor "telephone" games
		Play concentration games
Have students practice sequential counting of objects		Make up a new language

School Competencies: *Physical*

- Mobility
- Self-care
- Hand skills
- Strength
- Endurance

Suggested Activities:

Movement games that require postural changes • Cutting and pasting activities • Tracing • Sewing tasks • Pincer-grasp tasks such as those requiring the use of wooden clothes pins, keys and combination padlocks, shuffling cards, hide-in-your-hand games, pick-up sticks, using a spinning top to make designs • Hanging upsidedown off a chair and copying a design • Balance beams • Fishing for items using nets and magnets • Body extremity isolation games

Age 3	Age 4	Age 5
Keep it novel Keep it short-term Keep it fast-paced Use toys that are physically supported (e.g., tricycles instead of bicycles) Use scooter boards that are about the length of their bodies for hand/arm strengthening Do lacing tasks Cut "sunshines" and use play dough Play wikki stick games Use strawberry pickers to pick up discrete items and place in a specific spot	Use one roller skate to ambulate around a maze; allow one foot for stability on the floor, then expand task to use a buddy on carpet; keep nonskated foot up to be "pulled" for a few inches Do skateboard activities Use pedal-and-go toys or moon shoes to change balance Have students catch beanbags or balls while standing on an inner tube Have students practice combat crawling and/or isolation of upper or lower body for movement Do timed tasks/games	Play hanging games to incorporate kicking something or reaching out for something on an unstable surface Practice shoe tying Do lacing tasks that incorporate figure/ground discrimination Role play a time of day (e.g., pretend it's morning and teach a pal what to do) Have students cut out imbedded forms Do activities that require the crossing of the midline of the body (e.g., reaching across to get a needed supply)

School Competencies: *Intellectual*

- Performance task behaviors (rejection, motivation, curiosity, transitional skills, problem-solving, etc.)
- Time concepts (sequencing, getting work done on time, etc.)
- Task production (following directions: verbal, written, demonstrated, repeated, etc.)
- Retention (long-term vs short-term memory issues; ADD children)
- Task judgments (relies on teacher or peers/independent)
- Evaluation skills (accepting critical assessments, self evaluations).

Suggested Activities:

Sequential tasks that require students to make on-the-spot decisions that may or may not affect the outcome of the task • Prioritizing tasks from given reasons: give two directions one after the other—one to do now, one to do later—and tell them that you cannot repeat the directions, so they must listen carefully. Encourage "assists" such as picture-clues or assembled supplies. Establish criteria that they can grade themselves on.

AGE 3	AGE 4	AGE 5
Have two task "pods" where all the necessary supplies for a particular task are out and available; have students decide which pod they will go to first Keep activities to one or two repetitive steps Play discovery games for familiar items using clues Have treasure hunts Do timed tasks that have "stop" and "go" indicators throughout the activity Have each student tell a friend how to do something he or she was just taught	Increase the task "pods" to three Introduce two-step repetitive tasks Use transitions (e.g., finding a picture, cutting it out, pasting it, categorizing it) Use a timer with a bell or a beeper and make students start and stop at specific times; if they don't finish, have them think of ways they could have gotten the task done on time Think up ways to use a familiar item in an unfamiliar way	Keep the "pods" at three but make them multiple-step (three to four) Give students/groups a problem and ask them to find a solution (e.g., "You are a cave man and you need to build a hut, but hammers are not invented yet. How can you build a hut?") Have task carry over from one day to the next; have daily completion goals Do matching and sorting tasks in which students utilize similarities and differences Use picture directions and sequential picture cards to tell stories

Suggestions for Teachers: How to Have a Successful IEP Meeting

1. **Have the right mindset.**

   This meeting is your chance to show off your many teaching talents.

   Emphasize creativity.

   Your expertise is making familiar the unfamiliar to children.

2. **You are obviously not doing this for the money, so talk from the heart.**

   This is not about wanting to control.

   This is not about power.

   You have joys, fears, and dreams for the child. Talk about them.

   What are your joys? And your frustrations?

   What do you want from the child?

   Go in with a prepared list.

3. **You cannot help someone you do not like. So find something you like about the student and focus on it (even if this child agitates you).**

   Samples of statements that may correspond to your situation:

   Joys

   - He always greets you when he comes in the classroom.

   - He has something interesting to say.

   - He is artistic.

   - I can tell his mind is always working.

   - He is sensitive to others.

   - He has a sense of fair play.

   - He follows the rules and takes them seriously.

- He has a sense of community about other members of the class.

- He shares well.

- He is creative.

- His thoughts are often beyond his years.

- His thinking is often "outside the box." This can also be a frustration because it often confuses some more concrete children, which in turn complicates his social relationships.

Frustrations

- He doesn't complete his work on time.

- He sits fidgeting and wastes time.

- He doesn't seem to know when or how to ask for help.

- I can't figure him out.

- He seems to sabotage himself.

- He is disorganized, and no matter how many times I help him get organized, he can't keep up with any system consistently.

- He doesn't seem to understand the personal boundaries of the other children.

- He says things that are inappropriate.

- He tries too hard in social situations, and this turns off other kids.

- He has extreme reactions to corrective remarks.

- He doesn't seem to take responsibility for his work; he always has some excuse or another.

- I am afraid of hurting his feelings.

- He seems to get hurt easily.

- I feel he wants me to rescue him, and I don't know how.

- He doesn't stay on task.

- I am looking for suggestions on how to channel his positive qualities into the classroom.

- He is forgetful.

- He demands a lot of my time.

- He seems to need more stroking than other children.

Dreams:

(It is probably true that you and the parents share the *same dreams* and that all of you are worn out!)

- I want him to have friends.

- I want him to feel like he belongs at the school, like he has a niche here.

- I want him to feel like someone cares.

- I want him to feel that, despite his current level of functioning, someone has faith in him that he can make and reach his goals.

- I want him to feel he can exceed, succeed, and thrive.

- I want him to be confident in himself.

- I want him to feel connected to the learning process, the teachers, and the school.

- I want him to feel there is something special about him that is positive and unique.

- I want him to feel liked.

- I want him to be able to make the right choices in peer situations.

- I want him to know when and how to ask for help.

- I want him to know how to accept corrective remarks and how to reject ones that are not valid.

- I want him to know how to discriminate between potentially positive and negative situations.

- I want him to feel that he can try something slightly beyond his reach and that there are teachers here to help him.

- And when this growing up is over, I want him to be an independent, content, goal-directed, successful adult.

4. Now, as a team, think up ways the parents can help you and him reach these goals.

5. Set the IEP goals based on these dreams and fears.

6. Address the frustrations and let their resolution be part of the goal plan.

7. Give the parents specific things to do.

8. Establish a communication system so you can reach the parents quickly if you have questions or concerns (e.g., email, a communication book, etc.)

9. Everything should be in writing; keep a file. Have all persons present at the meeting sign the minutes.

10. Do not push for an IEP signature if the parents are hesitant or nervous.

11. You have the right to suggest that the meeting be reconvened, canceled, or adjourned if the tensions are too volatile. But first do everything to defuse the negativity.

12. Understand that an older child may want to be present. If you and the rest of the team don't want him present for the entire meeting, let him come in briefly either at the end or the beginning. Remember—he is the reason you are having this meeting.

FINAL NOTES

You are a teacher, not a genie. You are human. You have no magic wand; it is OK to say you need help. Benefit from the input of the parents; they are struggling too. Change takes effort. It can also be painful. You are aware of the ramifications of the struggles of children.

You are being *paid*. The parents are not your friends; they are not permanent in your life. This is your career. This is you and your professionalism on display. Be polite and keep focused on the goals. Get the parents on your "dream team." You are in the "successful kid business," so show off what you've got!

Everyone wins; you look great; the parents feel you are with them and that they are not swimming upstream; and the message to the child is one of caring and concern.

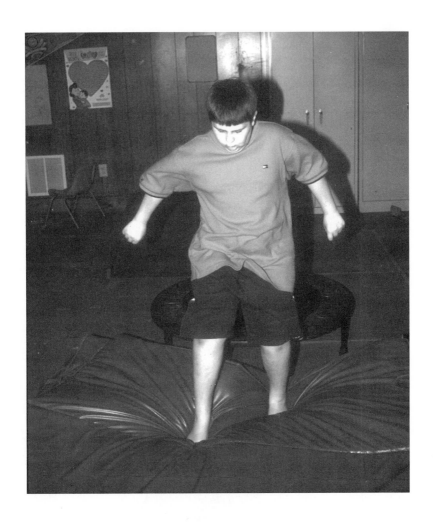

CHAPTER SEVEN

Occupational Therapy
in Action

The following photos are examples of occupational therapy in action.

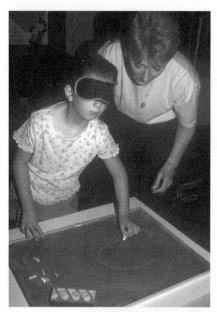 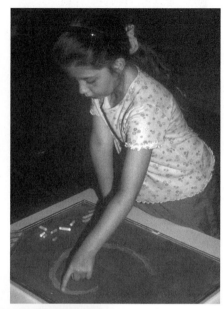

Promoting kinestatic
awareness.

Using Jan Olson's
Handwriting Without Tears.

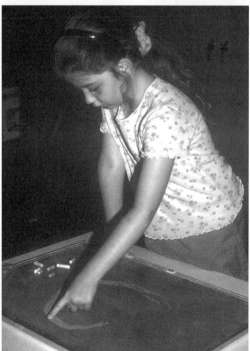

Magic C.

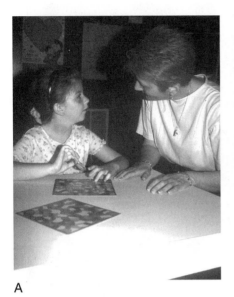 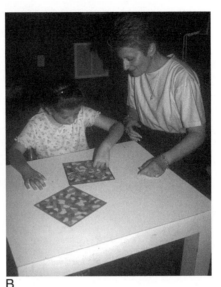

A B

Figure/Ground discrimination games.

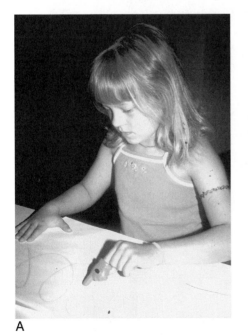 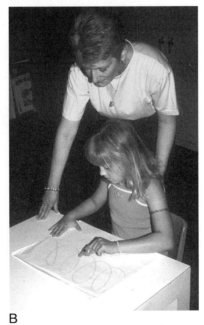

A B

Visual tracking.

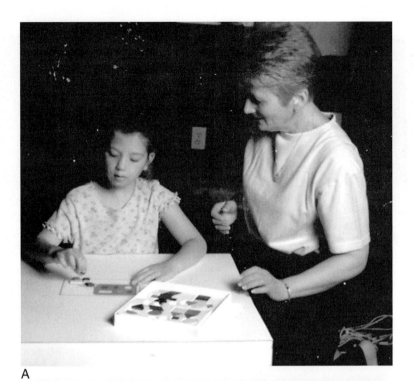

A

Part/Whole perception.

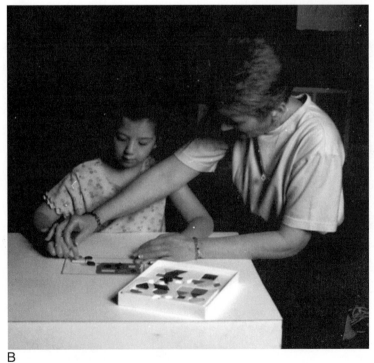

B

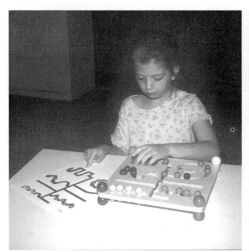

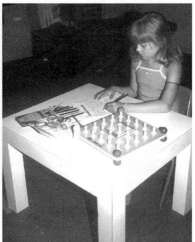

Design copy.

Using colored rubber bands.

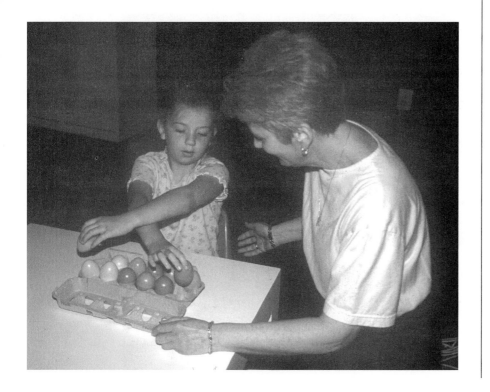

Plastic Easter eggs help teach students to cross the midline.

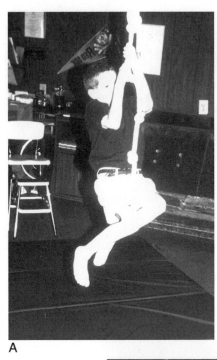

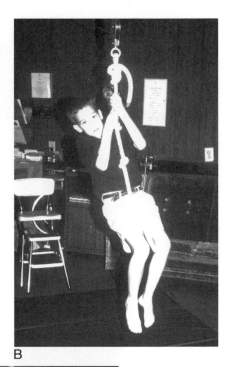

A

B

Fun on the zip line to increase upper body strength and stability.

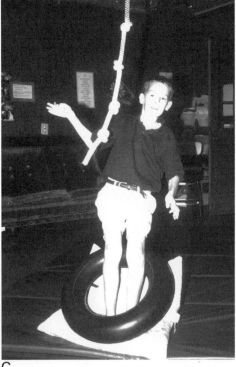

C

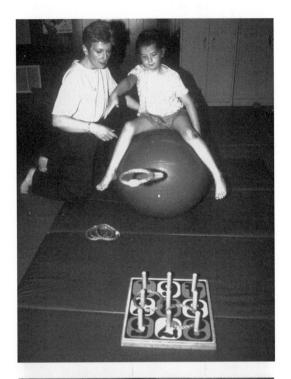

Insecure-balance postural adjustments.

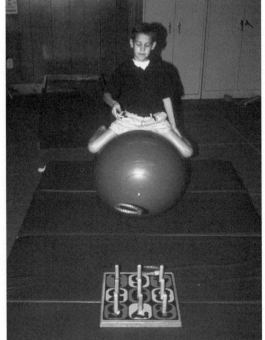

Secure-balance postural adjustments.

N o t e s

Combining motor planning
with visual pursuit.

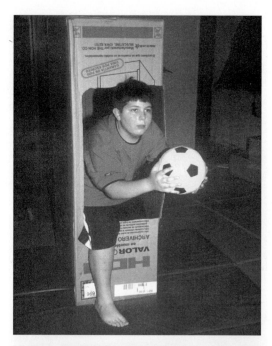

Mobility/stability with visual
motor tasks.

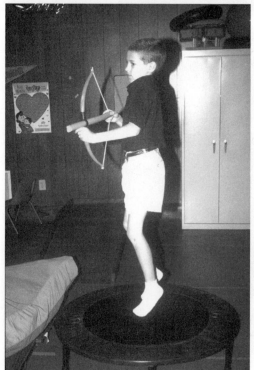

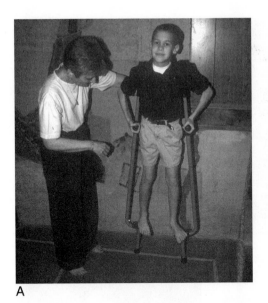

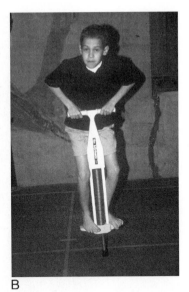

A

B

Weight shift and balance using stilts and pogo stick.

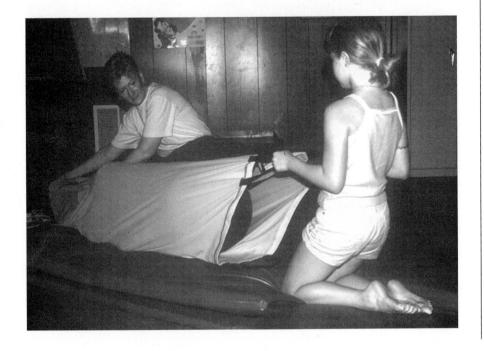

Movement through a sensory tunnel.

Perceiving body and space
with vision occluded using
southpaw tactile sock.

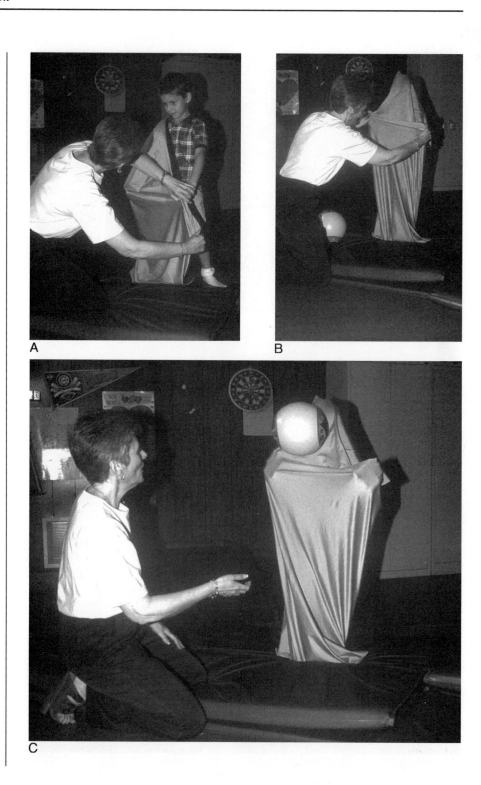

A

B

C

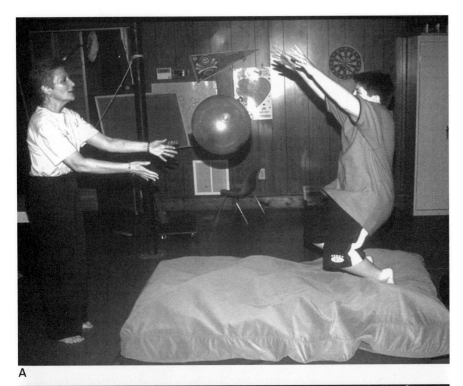

A

Learning to move and do at
the same time.

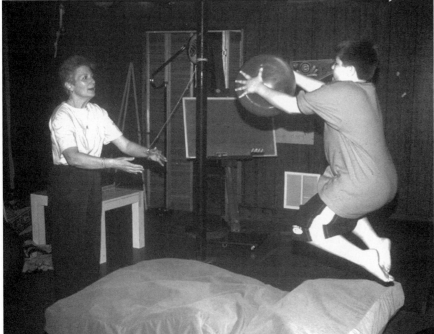

B

Using a flying turtle.

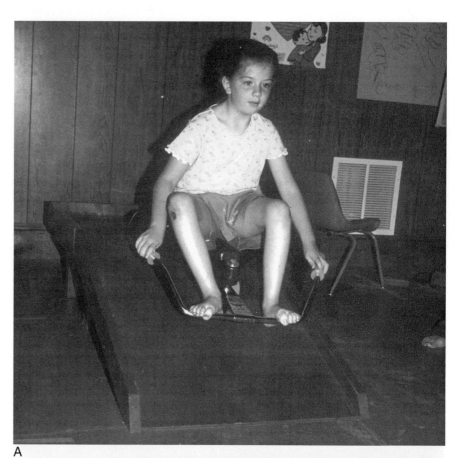

A

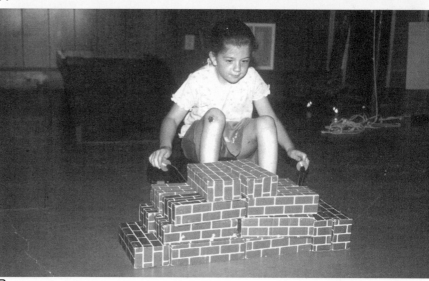

B

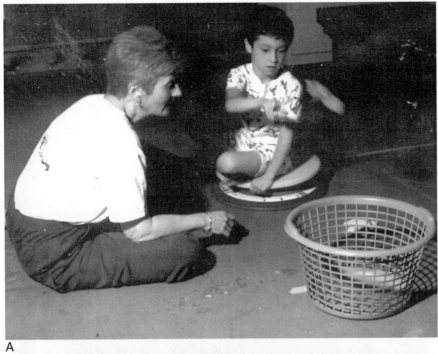

A

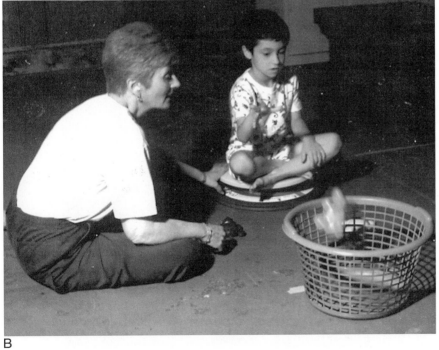

B

Crossing the midline. Note unstable pattern here.

A, Balance beam tracking.
B, Weight shift with
reaching and grasp-and-
release activities.

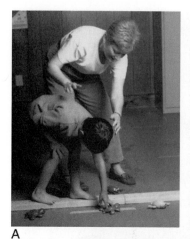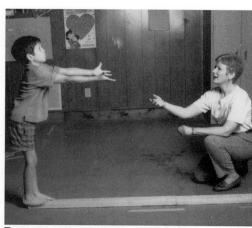

A

B

Falling from a zip line using
alternative postures.

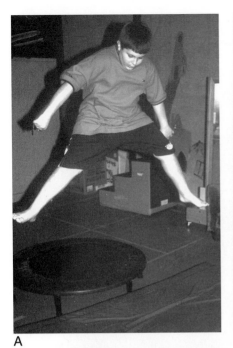

A

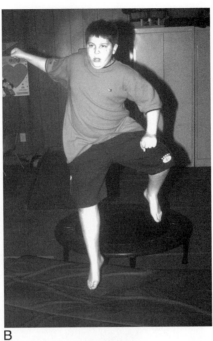

B

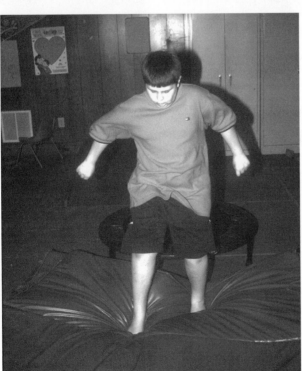

C

Developing body and space security and awareness.

Using southpaw crash mat to increase motor planning and secure/insecure extension.

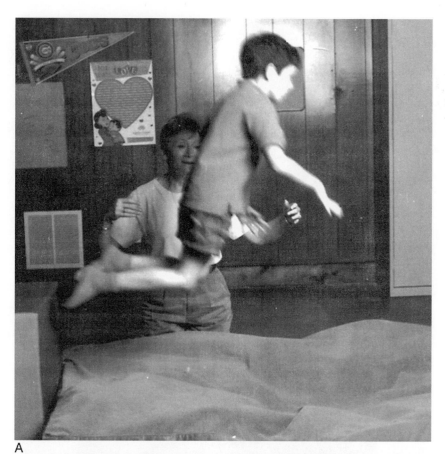

A

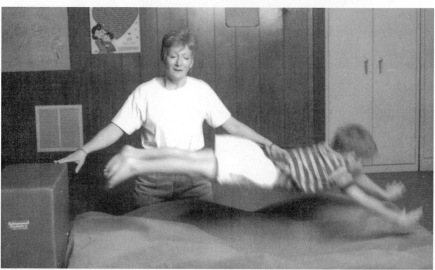

B

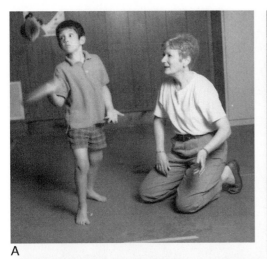

A

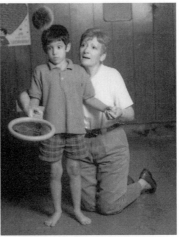

B

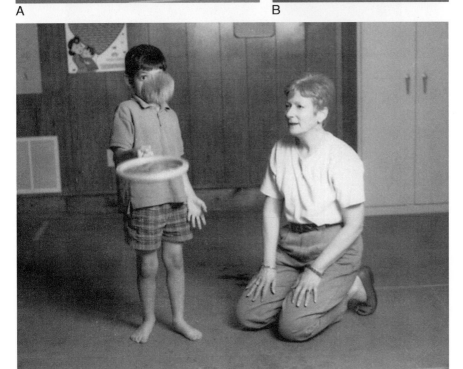

C

Right forearm rotation.

Stable balance and
co-contraction using
handled skate board.

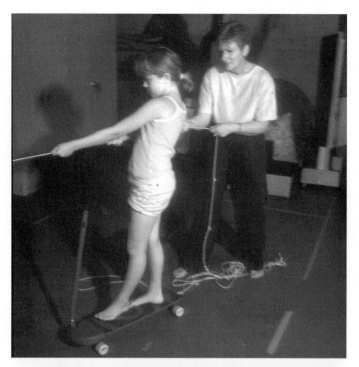

Unstable balance and co-
contraction using scooter
board.

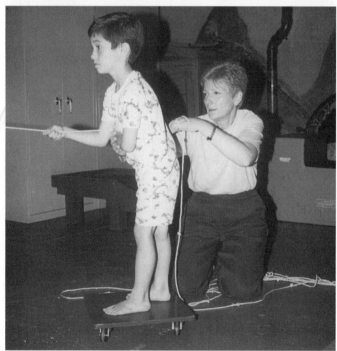

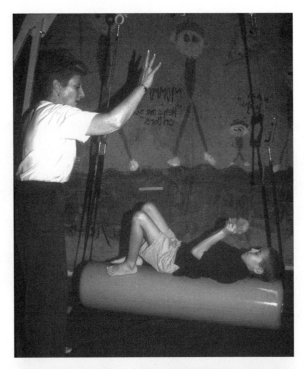

Postural adjustment.

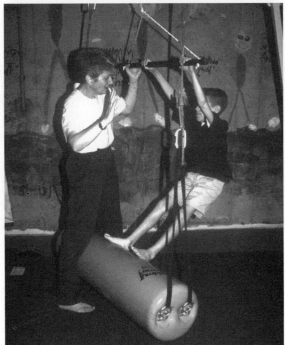

Combining motor planning with visual pursuit.

Balance and tracking.

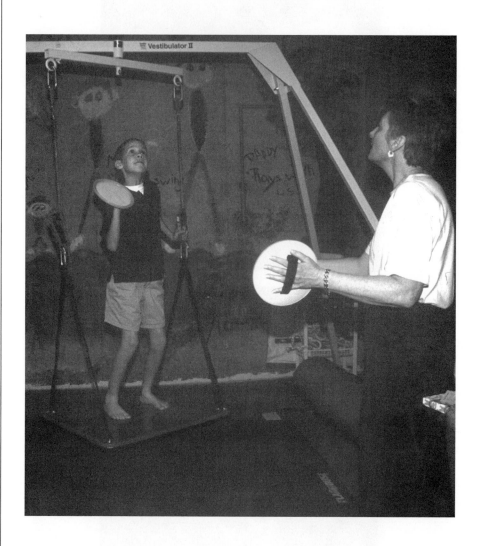

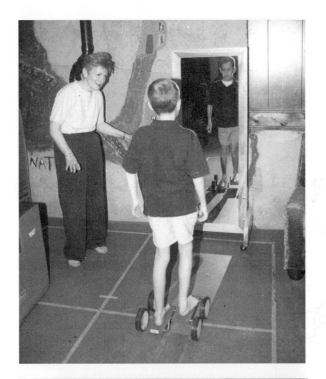

Using a pedal-and-go for weight shift, co-contraction, and mobility.

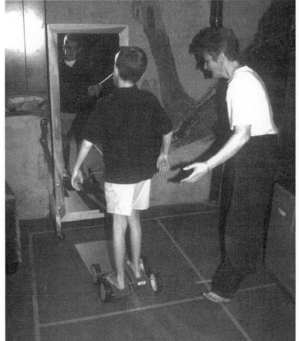

Mobility/stability with a visual target including reciprocal arm movements.

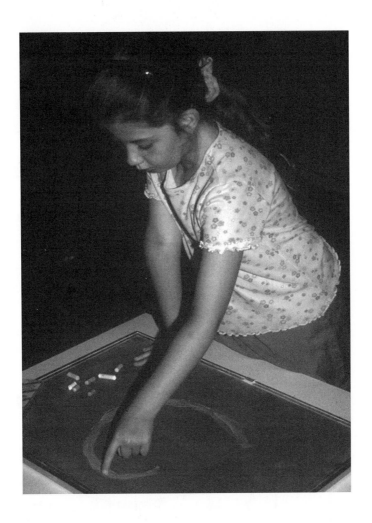

CHAPTER EIGHT

Student Writing Samples

My name is, _____.

Make a funny story.

    I felt _~~purpely~~_. I looked out of my window. A _ginger_ cow was coming along the street.

    "Hello," said the _happy_ cow. "I see you are _hungary_. I like people who are _green_ and have ~~hotel~~ hair."

    "Let's eat some _salty_ food," I said. "Then we can play _nosie_ games together." We did.

    "Where do you live?" I asked.

    "In a _upside-down_ ~~house~~," ~~said the~~ cow. "I must go home now."

    "Good-bye," I said. "Good-bye my ~~purpel~~ friend."

A, M.F. before therapy.

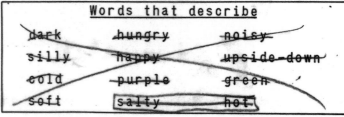

Words that describe

~~dark~~	~~hungry~~	~~noisy~~
silly	~~happy~~	upside-down
~~cold~~	~~purple~~	~~green~~
soft	salty	~~hot~~

Unit 5: Visualizing   81   Enrichment Activity

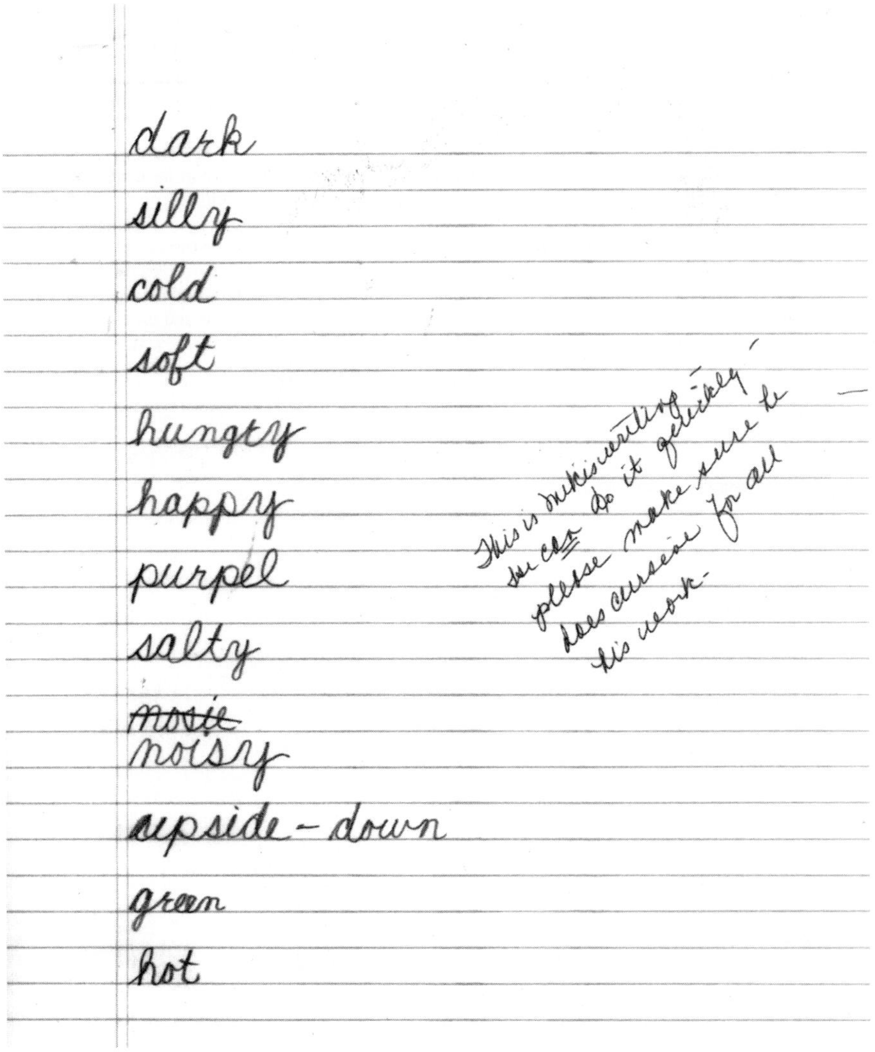

dark

silly

cold

soft

hungry

happy

purpel

salty

~~nosie~~

noisy

aepside – down

green

hot

This is intervirewriting / she can do it quickly / please make sure he / does cursive for all / his work –

B, M.F. after therapy.

Language Arts 7   Name
Mrs. Levine   Date

Letter to the Editor

Letters to the editor are written to express an opinion about a particular event or decision. Choose one of the stories from your anthology which deals with a controversial resolution, one upon which readers might have differing opinions. Write a letter to the editor, of at least four paragraphs in length, in which you express your opinion about how the conflict in one of your stories was resolved. Letters to the editor should be written in the first person (I). You should choose a resolution which you think was in some way unsatisfactory. Explain the conflict and resolution, and propose how the conflict might have been resolved more effectively. Fill in the worksheet below and use the notes to write your letter. You should include all of the information from your notes in the actual letter you will write.

Title and author: From Coffin To Rolls-Royce

List and describe the protagonists: Sandy Thomas

Describe the setting: World War II   Athens

A, M.S. before therapy.

Explain the conflict and what led up to it: he was in a coffen ~~and How he got out of it~~ How does he get out to a nertchral country

Explain how the conflict is resolved in the story: He reaches the nertchle country and He rids in a Rolls-Royce

Explain why this resolution is unsatisfactory: The car costs way to much to drive in after an escape

Describe a new and original resolution and explain why it would improve the story. A ride in a van because it makes more sense because a van costs less than a rolls-Royce

4/10/98

A B C D E F G H I J K L M N O P Q R S T U V W X Y

a b c d e f g h i j k l m n o p q r s t u v w x y z

abcde@ghijklmnopqrstuvwxyz

aBcD

aBcDeo

1 2 3 4 5 6 7 8 9 10 11 12 13 14 15 16 17 18 19 20

The astronauts flew past the moon

the astronaute

B, M.S. before therapy.
C, M.S. after therapy.

4/29/99

Before cursive my handwriting
looked real bad. Now it looks better
because of the cursive, It makes me
feel like I can get better grades.

Notes

A, A. before therapy.

B, A. after therapy.

7/9   C⁻

1. How is smoking bad for your Helth?
2. It damages the lungs and hart.
   Throat, mouth, eyes,
   It causes deadly diseses.
   What substance in cigrette smoke and cigrette bad fo
3. And substance in cigrette
   smoke are Tar, tobacco and Nicatin
   and carbon noxied monoxode
4. Why is it so hard to stop
   smoking?
   It is vey adtived to you what?
   It relaxes you of the
   carbon noxied

1. How is smoking bad for
   your health?

   It damages the lungs and heart.

   It causes deadly diseases.

   What substance in cigaretts
   are bad for you?

   The tar, tabacco, nicotine and
   carbon monoxide.

   Why is it so hard to stop
   smoking?

   It is very addictve to your
   body. It relaxes you because of
   the carbon monoxide.

A B E d e f g h

61.51% 0-20
A B C D E F G H I J K L M N
O P Q R S T U R W X Y Z

65.3% 0-6
a b c d e f g h i j k l m n o
p q r s t u v w x y z

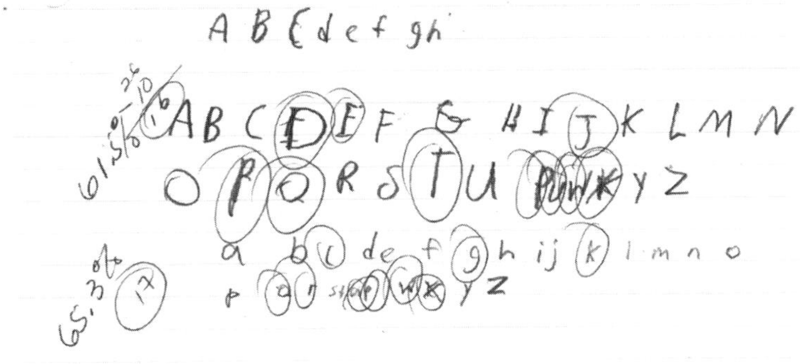

A, W. before therapy.

8/11/99

Dear Ms. Orloff,

I thank you for helping me write. It was

very fun.

from,

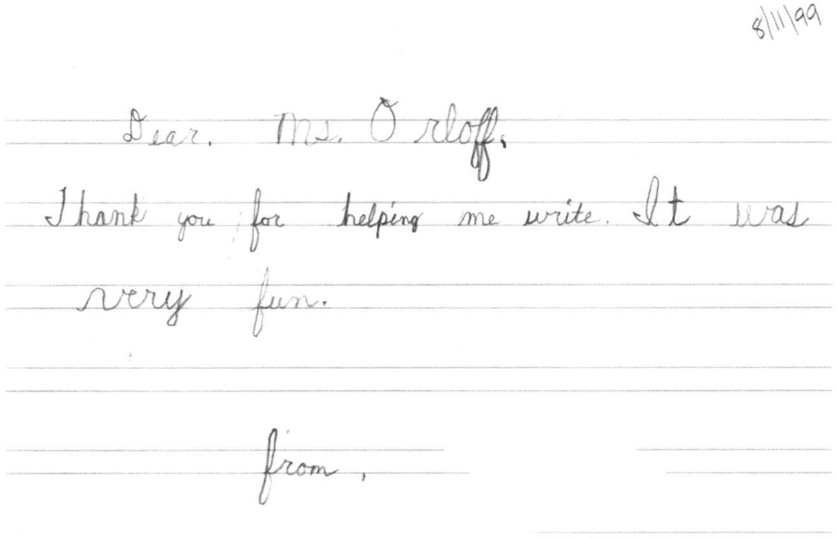

B, W. after therapy.

A, J. before therapy.

B, J. after therapy.

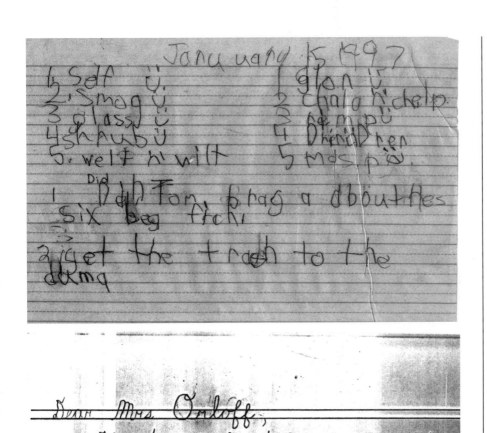

A, B. before therapy.

B, B. after therapy.

N o t e s

A, T. before therapy.

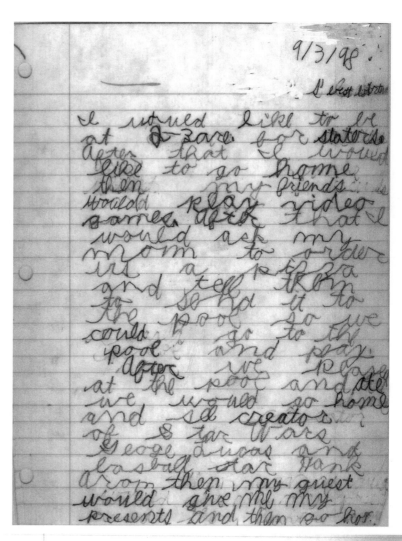

B, T. after therapy.

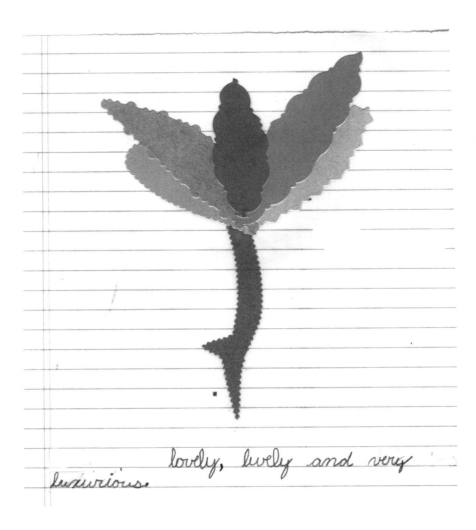

lovely, lively and very luxurious.

L. after therapy. L. destroyed all of her "befores," but was very proud of this.

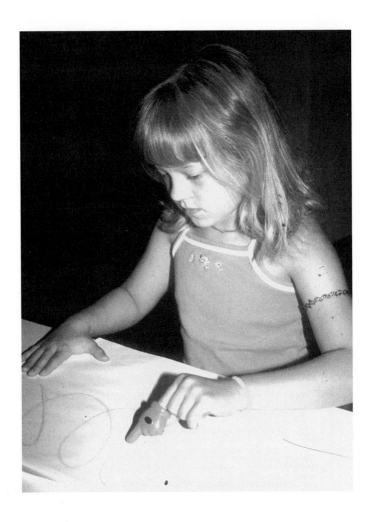

APPENDIX A

Function-based Glossary

Below is a glossary that has been developed to help parents and teachers understand common medical terms used to describe children seen by occupational therapists. Included for illustration are ways in which a child may manifest these issues, a few examples of occupational therapy interventions, and how those treatment activities change your child's related behaviors and performances.

Adaptation

Definition

Adaptation is the ability to translate the needs of a task into a pattern that is more functionally accessible to the child. Initially this is usually therapist facilitated; the goal is to enable the child to do this for herself.

Appearance

A child with an adaptation problem tends to be very literal and doesn't seem to be able to redirect her actions once she has started a task. She doesn't seem to "get it." She feels that just repeating a method that is not working will eventually make it work. Discovering alternatives is hard.

Intervention

Working from familiar to unfamiliar and building on familiar schemes to create new skills in unfamiliar situations; these activities are presented in both the fine and gross motor formats as well as manipulative- and cognitive-based formats.

Results

Child learns to become more independent and creative as well as less fearful of unfamiliar situations; oftentimes she is seen on the fringes of groups, and an increase in interactive responses is often noted.

ADD and ADHD

Definitions

ADD (attention deficit disorder) and *ADHD (attention deficit hyperactivity disorder)* refer to the inability to focus on a task for the required time without unusual "drifting" out of the task arena, including organization of the required assignment.

Appearance

This is the kid that the teacher tells you "needs to try harder," is "lazy," "can do it when he wants to," is "manipulative," etc. In reality, this is a kid who is scared, disorganized, at times obsessive (in an effort to overcompensate), and seems to have a hard time getting his homework started.

Intervention

Sensory-motor tasks that require different alert stages and "fidget" tasks that let the child cue into his own need to move and readjust; intricate tasks that require both decision-making and adaptive responses; gross motor obstacle courses; posturally challenging games.

Results

Self-regulation of movement needs; decreased moody responses; child seems more comfortable in his own skin; an understanding that he is ok, that he can be in charge of himself; that because he may not work as others do, he isn't "dumb."

ADL

Definition

ADLs (activities of daily living) are all tasks that are necessary for the maintenance of daily life, such as dressing, feeding, grooming, and initiating tasks.

Appearance

Children may reject tying shoes or take off their shoes by kicking them off while still tied. General appearance of the child and her organization of personal items may seem messy.

Intervention

Adaptive practice with the specific skills: organizing nonpersonal items in a game situation and figure/ground discrimination and in-hand manipulation games.

Results

Decreased rejection of self-care tasks and responsibilities; increased self-esteem; may develop a more relaxed response in social situations.

Apraxia

Definition

Apraxia is a disorder of voluntary movement, characterized by partial or complete incapacity to execute purposeful movements without impairment of muscular power or co-ordination.

Appearance

Children appear awkward or clumsy, most noticeably in large gross movements such as hopping and skipping. These kids seem to trip over nothing and bump into everything.

Intervention

Hitting a balloon up in the air; catching, kicking, and hitting balls in interactive games; problem-solving while going through an obstacle course.

Results

Increased ability to break down activities into manageable parts and problem-solve.

Co-contraction

Definition

Co-contraction is the ability of the muscles to hold a position, such as the muscle-man posture that little boys like to do.

Appearance

A child with a co-contraction problem may seem lethargic and "floppy." This situation is directly related to *tone,* which is the ability to hold a position against force; this is not the same as strength.

Intervention

Resistance play utilizing scooter boards, tug-of-war games, zip lines, prone swing activities, climbing activities, obstacle paths, moving, pushing, and pulling-in game situations.

Results

Child exhibits increased ability to sustain himself in a task game situation. This is most noticeable in gross motor situations but can also be seen in attention to directions and increased initiation of interactive activities with peers.

Cognitive Functions

Definition

There are two basic types of cognitive functions: automatic and cortical.

1. *Automatic functions* are learned habituated activities that can be done without a review of the process, hence the term *automatic*. An example of this would be writing one's name, tying shoes, etc.

2. *Cortical cognitive functions* are slow, deliberate, thoughtful movements. An example of this might be following directions for assembling an unfamiliar object.

Appearance

A child having difficulty with automatic responses approaches every task as something unfamiliar. This child seems to require more repetitions to imbed a rote task than other children do. She often presents as very cautious and fearful of making mistakes. She is literally thinking through every step of the required process even though she might have done the tasks before. A child experiencing difficulties in this area seems more dependent than her peers and is often reluctant to problem-solve within a given activity.

Another way to think about this is: automatic = fast, cortical = slow. We need both the fast and the slow systems for competent functional results. A child who is having difficulties with cortical functions is usually locked into the slow mode. Conversely, a child locked into the fast mode may appear impulsive and random in her responses. This looks like an ADD issue. A child without ADD will be able to "shift gears" easily to slow herself down; the child with ADD will require multiple interventions.

Interventions

For automatic functions: repetition of familiar tasks; presenting a familiar task and adding multiple unfamiliar components to it with step-by-step repetitions; "backward chaining" a task (instead of putting it together, take it apart step-by-step until you get to the beginning); doing tasks by feel rather than by sight.

For cortical functions: use a timer or a stopwatch and "beat your best time" with familiar and fun activities; establish organizational patterns to increase flow of tasks; use white noise to reduce distractions; give a chewable necklace to young children to alleviate the anxiety of being pushed to go faster.

Results

Increased task performance competency; smoother movements; easier response reactions in group situations; less anxiety in task demand situations; decreased resistance to unfamiliar tasks; increased willingness to enter into unfamiliar situations; increased pride in finished assignments.

Flexion and Extension Patterns

Definition

Extension and flexion patterns are the ability to come into and away from the body in both static (co-contracted/holding) and dynamic (movement/fluidity) modes.

Appearance

The child with poor flexion/extension patterns may have difficulty catching a ball because he stabilizes his arms with his elbows close to his body, or his posture may appear round-shouldered, and sitting straight in a chair is a posture that cannot be sustained. In addition, this child often has difficulty with weight shift from one side of the body to the other, as well as reaching across the midline of his body. He also tends to hold and write with the same hand.

Intervention

Stretching and pulling activities on the stomach, such as scooter boards; extension in a net swing; standing on a moving bolster; weight-shift activities on a tilt board; games while sitting on a one-legged stool; moving hands through a resistance (play dough, weighted box, etc.); placement precision tasks that require stability on one side and movement on the other (usually dominant) side.

Results

More relaxed performance styles in both the gross and fine motor realms; less fidgety when sitting in a chair; increased ability to enter into interactive games with peers; increased self-esteem (he is not averting others, but meeting them face-to-face); increased postural stability; more fluid range of movements; increased willingness to try unfamiliar tasks; and when combined with a graded writing program, greatly improved handwriting!

Grasp

Definition

The ability to grasp a necessary object is most often used in reference to a style in which the child holds a pencil and/or utensils. The basic styles are palmar (using the whole hand); static (over stabilized, rigid, intense); and dynamic (relaxed, movement-oriented, fluid). There are many variations of grasp within these categories; these are broad descriptions.

Appearance

Poor grasp is often what a teacher identifies in students with poor handwriting and/or an inability to tie their shoes. The teacher may not be astute enough to look at the problem's precursors (flexion/extension, tone, etc.), but sees a stressed grasp, slow production, sloppy work (often relegated as "not trying"), and/or incomplete assignments. This is when a child is sent to the occupational therapist to "fix" the handwriting. Parents and teachers do not initially understand that this is a motor relearning process that is not done in two to three sessions, but gradually over time (several months or more depending upon the severity).

Intervention

Pick-up Stix, dominoes, or lacing activities; using strawberry pickers or tweezers to put and place things; rubber band designs on a raised peg board; games with magnets of different sizes and strengths; sewing; various arts and crafts activities; stability/mobility patterns that facilitate holding on the nondominant side so that the dominant side can move (remember that stability comes before mobility developmentally, so in order to write, which is movement, stability must be a secure posture).

Results

Confidence; pride in self and work; ownership of things they do and make in school; signing their names to their work so that everyone sees who made it, not just the teacher who has learned to decipher their (non)styles; increased self-care abilities; improved grooming habits; less sloppiness when eating; more thoughtful execution of required tasks; increased competencies and independence with school and home assignments.

Hypotonic/Hypertonic

Definitions

Not to be confused with strength (power), *tone* is co-contraction of muscles over time to hold a functional position. One's endurance is directly related to one's tone. A child who is hypotonic (undertoned) is loose, wiggly, and unstable. A child who is hypertonic (overtoned) is extreme, tense, and overstabilized.

Appearance

A hypotonic child seems to "poop out" quickly; his writing is usually very light, and related skills such as coloring and cutting reflect this instability, looking "wispy" in nature. A hypertonic child looks like a robot—stiff and unbending, with clenched hands. Fine motor skills are also affected since most of his energy is used keeping himself steady. His handwriting is very pressured and jerky, and he will admit that writing makes his hand hurt.

Intervention

Whole-body approach, for not just the tone of the hands needs to be normalized, although it is in the hands that hypotonicity and hypertonicity become the most obvious; multiple weight-bearing activities; hanging from zip lines; pulling back on a large Nerf shooter; skating; and pushing a heavy basket from place to place. For the hands, cutting resistive surfaces such as play dough and cardboard; using strawberry pickers to pluck small beads from a dough or Styrofoam ball; finger cymbals.

Results

When tone is brought into functional ranges, total body movement becomes more fluid. Hypotonic kids are noted to play more in gross motor activities; hypertonic kids are noted to be able to relax more, go to sleep easier, and frustrate less automatically. Fine motor skills including but not limited to handwriting markedly improve, as do most dressing, grooming, and other self-care skills.

Kinesthesia

Definition

Kinesthesia is the ability to have an internal body map that alerts and directs you through space. This is the ability to get from your car to your back door in the dark or from your bed to the bathroom in the middle of the night without turning on a light; you "know" the path.

Appearance

A child with a kinesthesia problem always seems to be bumping into things; she continually has a "lost" look about her. Sending her to the office (in school) or to her room to get something often takes much longer than anticipated, and she is often accused of dawdling. She "lands" at a new destination almost every time she leaves her stability point (e.g., class seat, space in front of the TV, etc.), and often she can appear somewhat ritualistic (e.g., having to always sit in the same spot in the car).

Intervention

Touch activities with a variety of textures, densities, shapes, and positions; blindfolded games; games in novel spaces (e.g., in oddly shaped boxes, under tables, etc.); doing a pattern first with vision and then without to stimulate internal memory of a particular pattern; internal visualization games (with vision occluded) (e.g., "Imagine in your mind a circle. Draw one as you walk on the floor. Now remembering where your circle is, come over to the side of the room and place in your circle three things.") (can also be used as a desktop activity).

Results

More secure movement patterns; increased efficiency in tasks; faster response time when asked to do something; increased willingness to enter into unfamiliar situations; increased ability to enter into tasks in which immediate success is not guaranteed; increased agility; enhanced repertoire of "preferred" games, sports, etc.; less "loner" behavior; diminished "clinging" behaviors. In general, she becomes less tied to her immediate world, gaining confidence in her internal environmental security.

Long-term and Short-term Memory

Definition

Long-term and short-term memory are actually two separate functions, controlled by two separate areas of the brain. Short-term memory accounts for about 80% of our memory and is the reason we can remember details for a test and then be unable to recall them an hour later. Long-term memory is a more complex process and actually holds less information than the short-term centers but is considered permanent, which is why people with Alzheimer's disease can speak of the past so clearly.

Appearance

When a parent asks a child on Tuesday, "Do you have any homework?" he may answer "no," not because he is avoiding responsibility, but because he honestly doesn't remember until a peer asks him how a project or assignment is going. Parents and teachers see the panic phase and the child gets labeled "Johnny come lately" when he is honestly lost. Many children with learning problems have just the reverse memory of the average population. Their long-term abilities to keep data are superior, but in many cases they have significantly impaired short-term memories. Complicated by the fact that many of these kids are very bright, they look like they are being defiant, lazy, and uninvolved, when the truth is that they cannot remember instructions for new tasks because the instructions are stored in the short-term centers. Therefore in order to learn something new, these children appear as if they are obsessively repeating something, when in fact they are memorizing the needed information.

Intervention

Learning the sequences to novel games and activities; obstacle courses; and strategy games such as checkers, chess, and Connect Four can be nonthreatening activities to develop alternative patterns that will be less cumbersome than the multiple repetitive techniques most commonly used. By taking a familiar game and changing the rules, the child must adapt his thinking to participate. These types of tasks are often used simultaneously with other tasks for other goals such as sequencing and organization skills.

Results

Fewer last-minute "rush hour" projects; new strategies help avoid these pitfalls, but they must be learned in an orderly sequential program of graded activities. It is a rare child who can learn this on his own.

Motor Planning

Definition

Motor planning is the coordination of the brain and the body to produce smooth, purposeful, successful movements.

Appearance

A child with motor planning problems is your typical klutz. She wants to get to *B* but doesn't know how to get off *A*. She is often labeled *passive aggressive* when she is not dawdling, but truly lost.

Intervention

Multiple gross and fine motor games to increase automatic repertoire of responses that will fit into a new situation with minimal adaptation. Task problem-solving and other (diminishing) supported tasks.

Results

Increased self-confidence; the ability to participate in unfamiliar situations; improved peer relationships, because now she can be counted upon in a group to do what she is assigned or has volunteered to do.

Muscle Tone

Definition

Muscle tone is the ability of a specific group of muscles to co-contract and stabilize for the purpose of a sustained movement. Writing is a prime example of a task that requires both stability and mobility (e.g., taking notes, taking a test, etc.) over time.

Appearance

A child with muscle tone problems appears to fatigue easily and have primarily short-term endurance and is not seen using recess to run around. He often picks a buddy to walk and chat with and then feels rejected when that friend also wants to go off and run. Pencil grasp is either too intense (in an effort to compensate) or too fragile.

Intervention

Various activities include both gross and fine motor patterns. Stability comes outward from the center of the body, so securing trunk stability is the first step. This can be done in many ways: games in a resistance tunnel; scooter boards; tug-of-war; skating; games that require the lifting and moving of weighted objects and in-hand manipulative skills.

Results

Improved manual dexterity; increased ability to maintain an appropriate "alert" phase so that attention issues often diminish; improved cutting and writing skills; increased speed in completing familiar tasks; enhanced affective responses.

Nystagmus

Definition

Nystagmus is the reflex reaction of the eyes to movement. After the child is spun or rotated, there should be a noticeable excursion and duration of eye fluctuation. The fluctuation is stimulated by the semicircular canals of the inner ear and lets us know "which end is up."

Appearance

Children with a depressed or absent nystagmus may not exhibit any superficially remarkable behaviors, but when parents are questioned, these are the kids that love amusement parks and can enjoy all the rides many times. This intense movement stimulates those "sleeping" reflex centers (vestibular system), and the movement, which could easily make others sick, is soothing to them.

Intervention

Graded by intensity, duration, speed, and direction, initiate movement activities on a variety of surfaces that challenge children's sense of gravity and promote an increased awareness of their bodies in space. These kids need supervision at play because they can become thrill seekers in an effort to provide their systems with the stimulation they are craving.

Results

Decreased restless behaviors; normalization of muscle tone; increased visual tracking; increased attention; increased ability to make postural changes as needed; increased stability/mobility patterns; normalization of tactile (touch) responses; less distraction by extraneous stimuli.

Prone and Supine

Definitions

Prone and *supine* refer to specific body positions. Someone who is prone is lying on his stomach; someone who is supine is lying on his back. Stability/mobility patterns occur in both positions, so it is important to develop both. They can exist exclusively of each other.

Appearance

A child with stability/mobility problems in the prone and/or supine positions has no overtly defining characteristics. Deficits in this area are discernible only upon specific testing. However such deficits can impede success at sports and may contribute to random fatigue responses. Rejection of these positions can also be related to the tactile system, so activities stress the synergistic relationship between movement and touch.

Intervention

Play/pretend swimming in a "tactile box"; Twister-like games, etc.

Results

More agility and flow of movements; less ritualistic behaviors (e.g., he doesn't always have to have a special chair when watching TV and his body can now adapt to a variety of positions comfortably).

Proprioception

Definition

Proprioception is the internal awareness of the body and its specific parts (muscle, bone, joints, etc.) that allow for postural security and position in space. It is important as a precursor to all purposeful movements. It is the proprioceptive feedback that allows us to make postural changes and adjustments as needed.

Appearance

A child with proprioceptive difficulties is often described as a "Jell-O" kid because she looks firm but is really shaky. She cannot navigate from one place to another in smooth fluid movements; she has a lot of stop-and-go qualities to her habituated responses. She is constantly shifting from one position to another, seeking out a comfort zone she cannot find because her system cannot locate where she is and what body part is needed to make the adjustments.

Intervention

Resistance activities with movement such as Simon Says and Mother May I?; balance beams and ramp activities; holding various dissimilar shapes and weights in each hand; moving through an obstacle course wearing/carrying novel objects of varying weights and degree of obstruction to movement; activities that incorporate kinesthetic responses; games played with sight and movement occluded.

Results

Increased control over her own body; more secure movement patterns; the ability to discern when a postural adjustment needs to be made and to what degree; less random wavering of body in an attempt to maintain positional neutrality and stability.

Sensory Modulation

Definition

Sensory modulation is ostensibly a reflexively self-regulated ability of the body to adjust to changes in sensory stimuli (e.g., moving away from too much noise, steadying oneself on a rocking boat, ignoring a scratchy sweater in order to pay attention to a cognitively demanding task, etc.).

Appearance

A child with sensory modulation difficulties often looks out of control; he moves in extremes. It is as if he is on "high alert"— visually, auditorily, emotionally. He has difficulty finding a middle ground and is usually emotionally sensitive; he often requires significant external support to maintain control.

Intervention

Multiple activities that incorporate the discrimination of two or more sensory stimuli in order to complete the required task (could include combinations of sound and touch or of smell and visual discrimination).

Results

The ability to maintain a reasonable work pace with interference; less frustration; fewer outbursts; less anger in task situations; increased control over emotions; increased tolerance of unfamiliar tasks; heightened awareness of internal mood shifts; the acquired ability to make appropriate changes in anticipation of need.

Sensory Registration

Definition

Sensory registration is the ability to receive and catalogue incoming stimuli so that appropriate reactions and actions may take place. It is the degree to which we can be our own "biofeedback" machines so we can recognize when the sensory input is appropriate or noxious.

Appearance

Children who have deficits in their sensory registration are known to overreact or underreact to specific stimuli. For example, a child who is hit by another child in the lunch line may perceive a punch when he was only slightly bumped. Another may not feel how hot a burner is in the chemistry lab, and so forth.

Intervention

Games that require the discrimination and classification of specific stimuli; changing "What's my line?" to "What's my sensory system?" allows the child in a risk-free environment to experiment with various sensory situations and consider possible solutions.

Results

Less volatility; more personal responsibility; increased comfort in unpredictable situations; increased experimentation in unfamiliar task scenarios; increased anticipation of possible personal needs in a specific set of circumstances.

Stability/Balance

Definitions

The laws of development are that before one can move, one must first become stable; one must have a secure starting point. For children, this is rocking on all fours, the prewalking weight-bearing that gives them the foundation, or balance, for movement.

Stability is central, from the trunk of the body, whereas balance involves the whole body and incorporates tone, flexion, extension, motor planning, proprioception, and kinesthesia. Walking toddlers are an example of movement before secure stability. They move with their legs farther apart and arms stiff and outstretched; they are prepared to fall.

Appearance

A tightrope walker moves by holding a long balancing stick; a child with a stability/balance problem walks using everything she has. She is usually stiff, with clenched fists and jerky movement. As she grows, she is habitually stiff. One example of this is poor handwriting in school. She tries to hold the paper and write with one hand and support her body with the other.

Intervention

Activities that require both stability and mobility for successful completion, such as lying prone on a platform swing and stopping herself with her nondominant hand and stacking cones or picking up a puzzle piece with the other; roller skating games; scooter activities; skateboarding; balance beam games; games that require her to start motionless, perform a specific motor task, return to a motionless position, and repeat the pattern. She may be a good soccer player because she is always on the move but cannot play basketball or baseball as well because these sports require starting and stopping.

Results

Fewer sedentary activities; more participation in group games; improved handwriting; increased organizational abilities; less frustration. In other words, this is a child who is now in the driver's seat whereas before, the car (i.e., body) was driving her, and she was stiff, holding on for dear life to compensate for insecure stability and balance mechanisms.

Strength/Endurance

Definitions

Strength is the actual amount of force the body is able to exert in order to lift, move, or place something. *Endurance* is the length of time this activity can be sustained.

Appearance

A child with good strength but poor endurance works in bursts with significant "downtime." In this case, other sensory-motor factors are influencing the child's ability to stay on task. Strength can occur without endurance, but endurance rarely exists without strength.

Intervention

Weight-bearing games; wheelbarrow walking with specific placement tasks required; scooter board games; timed activities (a personal "beat the clock"); multi-tasking several activities that require weight shifting, gross motor alteration, and fine motor alteration.

Results

Increased participation; assignments done with less procrastination (which was really the need to regroup because the child ran out of steam).

Symmetrical/Asymmetrical

Definitions

Symmetrical movement ocurs when both sides of the body are moving together (synchronization). An example of this would be both arms flexed at the same time. *Asymmetrical* movements, the opposite of symmetrical movements, are what we normally do automatically. We walk swinging our arms back and forth; children skip; we hold on to the counter when we have to get something almost out of our reach, and one foot may bear all our weight when we do this.

Appearance

A child with symmetrical movements is a "bullet" kid. She moves as a single unit with little or no reciprocal pattern, usually in very stiff postures, in either a full-speed-ahead or a full-stop mode. Sometimes it is much more subtle. She can appear as if nothing is wrong, and then little things get snagged, like handwriting, math papers, precise agility in sports (she can play well, but she is usually in the offensive position).

Intervention

Vestibular swing activities; using the platform to be prone to push and fixate while completing another task; weight shift games on the holster swing; moving the holster in a circle by just shifting her body; pulling herself hand-over-hand along a designated path wearing in-line skates; painting, doing a puzzle, or making a Lite Brite pattern while standing with one foot on the other and one arm on the table for stability; jumping from one foot to the other on a trampoline.

Results

Less rigidity of movements; more willingness to try unfamiliar tasks; reduced fear of falling; increased scanning abilities; normalization of body tone; increased ability to focus on task without holding herself steady.

Transitional Activities

Definition

Transitional activities are the tasks that help us go from one situation to another. It's like an automatic "pre-1st" (a grade in some school systems for children who have completed kindergarten but are not quite ready for 1st grade) for our bodies; we are not quite ready for a big move, so we take a little one instead.

Appearance

Children who find it hard to transition from one task to another often fixate on the task at hand, sometimes obsessively. They resist any changes in their lives and react strongly to externally imposed changes. In toddlers this can be observed in the child who rejects all toys but one type (e.g., dinosaurs), refuses to greet any unfamiliar people even with parental support, and seldom initiates interactive play unless in a totally familiar environment.

Intervention

Structured sessions with choices, with noted beginnings and endings to all discrete tasks; increasing their comfort zone of change by slowly decreasing the amount of advance warning when a project is about to end and another begin; stopping a task midway through to go on to something else and then coming back to it later (this can be done in many activities: building a cardboard box house, papier-mâché, puzzle creations, etc.).

Results

Decreases situational anxiety; increased ability to think through tasks and to reduce them into component parts to be able to self select points at which the task may be stopped and resumed later; increased acceptance and interest in a variety of toys; less fearfulness of new situations and people; increased problem-solving skills.

Vestibular Stimulation

Definition

Vestibular stimulation is the fluid movement in the semicircular canals of the ear that triggers eye movement, tactile perception, balance, midline, and gravitational and vibratory responses in each of us. It is our "putting it all together" system. It takes all of the above mentioned sensations and movements and signals them to create the movement desired. It is our "this end is up" alert system.

Appearance

Children with vestibular problems usually fall into two major categories: those with too little stimulation and those with too much. The kids with too little are your "roller coaster forever" kids; they never seem to get dizzy, and they are always on the move because the stimulation is comforting for them. What adults feel when their ears are stopped up, these children feel in their whole bodies. For kids with too much stimulation, any movement makes them sick. They are your "sitters"; they want to be still.

Intervention

For the kids with too little stimulation, the more spinning, moving, up-ending activities the better. For the kids with too much stimulation, a slow program of graded movement activities that will expand their tolerance and acceptance of movement is recommended. Use skate boards, scooters, scooter boards, games on ramps, obstacle courses that require positional shifts, etc.

Results

Increase in accuracy of all tasks that require the utilization of both sides of the body; improved reading (both eyes), walking (both feet), eating, dressing, and playing; increased ability to tolerate, anticipate, and eventually welcome novel movement experiences; decreased exaggerated tonal responses; increased fine motor skills including handwriting.

Vision/Perception

Definition

Vision is only visual acuity—how far and near you can see with and without correction (i.e., glasses or contact lenses). *Perception* is translating that acuity into meaningful symbols, organizing them, and reorganizing them for problem-solving; task attack skills; and discrimination. There are seven realms of perception: visual discrimination, visual memory, visual-spatial relationships, visual form constancy, visual sequential memory, visual figure/ground, and visual closure.

Appearance

Children with vision/perception problems are often your "homework war" kids. Every piece of work looks like hieroglyphics to them, and so they habituate a fight-or-flight reflex and come up with a thousand reasons not to get to the task. This is often interpreted as avoidance; sometimes these kids are labeled *passive-aggressive* when all they really are is scared. Children may have some, but rarely do they have all, of these systems impaired. Standardized testing is the only way to discern which realms are strong and which are weak.

Intervention

By capitalizing on the stronger realms and helping the child feel successful, the therapist can help transform these deficits into positive tools for increased function. Some activities involve paper and pencil, but many involve gross motor manipulation as well.

Results

Decreased fear; more compliance with assigned chores; increased organization; decreased rejection of required work; increased security in social situations; increased problem-solving; ability to use familiar skills to complete unfamiliar tasks. The child will have learned to transform a misperception into something meaningful and functional, and as they feel more secure in the world, they become more socially at ease.

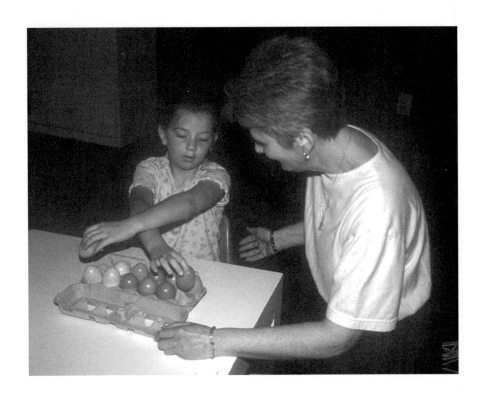

APPENDIX B

What Does Uncle Sam Say About
All of This?

There are primarily four laws that directly impact services delivered to learners who have a diagnosis of a specific learning disability.

1. Individuals with Disabilities Educational Act (IDEA), Public Law 94-142 initially was passed in 1975 and is reauthorized every 5 years.

2. Americans with Disabilities Act (ADA), Public Law 101-336 was passed in 1990 and provides accommodations for children who have a diagnosis of a specific learning disability.

3. Section 504 of the Rehabilitation Act of 1973, Public Law 93-112.

4. Educational Act, Public Law 94-142, Part B provides mandatory services for children 3 to 21 years, and Public Law 99-457 provides discretionary state services for children 0 to 5. Early intervention programs are delivered through the latter program.

IDEA

This law incorporates the learning situation with defined transition services as "...free and appropriate education . . . a coordinated set of activities for a student, designed within an outcome-oriented process . . . which promotes movement from school to post-school activities including post-secondary education, vocational training, integrated employment, including supported employment, continuing adult education, adult services, independent living or community participation. The coordinated set of activities shall be based upon the individual student's needs, taking into account the student's preferences and interests and shall include instruction, community experiences, employment development, and other post-school adult living objectives, and when appropriate acquisition of daily living skills and functional vocational evaluation." (20 U.S.C. § 1401 [a][l 9])

In 2003, the IDEA was recertified by the US House of Representatives, and at the time of this writing was yet to be ratified by the US Senate. However some very important changes were made in both the content and intent of this law. It is known as *HR 1350*. Perhaps the best way to understand a few of the major changes in this law would be in tabular form:

Summary of IDEA Standards

Original IDEA (1970)	Revised IDEA, 2003 (passed in the US House of Representatives, 2003)
IEP meetings to assess goals and program will be held yearly.	IEP meetings will be scheduled every 3 years, though parents can request one at any time. This significantly reduces paperwork for teachers.
A 20-point difference between performance and verbal scores on psychoeducational evaluations can qualify a student for special services as a child with a "learning disability."	Eliminated—This is no longer a criterion for identifying children. No eligibility documents are needed. New criteria: "failure to learn in traditional settings" (this is a subjective judgment call).
Learning disabilities are labeled as *disabilities*.	*Learning disabilities* are labeled as *mild disabilities*. (The national Division for Learning Disabilities, a subgroup of the National LD Association, stated, "We believe that LD is not a 'mild' disability but rather a serious, significant and often severe disability that pervades many parts of a person's life. And it is life long." [Division for Learning Disabilities: DLD testimony on IDEA reauthorization, *DLD Times* 20:3 Winter, 2003.])
IDEA was fully funded.	IDEA revisions were to be linked with full funding. The new bill has no provision to ensure that additional resources will be provided.
A student could not be expelled for behaviors associated with a learning disability.	HR1350 (the revised IDEA) allows for students to be expelled unilaterally and placed in an alternative setting for any violation of the school's code of conduct, including chewing gum, shouting in class, or having a plastic fork in their lunch bags. This means, for example, a child with Tourette's syndrome could be expelled for shouting, even though it is a result of his disability.
There was no gag rule.	New provision states that employees of parent centers and their affiliates would lose all federal funding as a result of engaging in "any legislative advocacy activity on behalf of students with disabilities and their families."
IEP goals included long- and short-term objectives.	Short-term objectives are eliminated. The school district is responsible for establishing alternative testing and assessment methods.
Parent(s) could file due process claims.	Statute of limitations on due process: new law bars parent(s) of LD child from filing due process claims for the issues related to problems more than a year before the claim. This limits the parents in using school performance histories to support their request for services and supports.
There were no waivers for compliance.	"10 State Waiver Demonstration Project" allows for the Secretary of Education to waive IDEA statutory and regulatory provisions without recourse.

The main advocate for a child is his or her parent. That is why it is essential that parents know the laws and understand them completely. (Copies of all laws are available by writing to the government printing office in Pueblo, Colorado.) To assist with interpretation of the laws specific to the IDEA, there is a website that can be of benefit: http://edworkforce.house.gov/democrats/ideaform.html.

Keeping up with the laws while holding down a job, raising children, and keeping a family functioning is overwhelming. Wheelchairs and crutches gain sympathies that brains do not. Learning disabilities, for the most part, cannot be seen. Children with learning disabilities, left unidentified or with inadequate services, often become the outcasts at school. It is incumbent upon the parent to ensure that the school is providing their LD child with free and appropriate education.

Americans with Disabilities Act

The ADA, passed in 1973, states that students with disabilities should have full access to public facilities including school, gym, and playground. It goes further to state that "full access" also includes the attainment of intellectual data (i.e., the classroom). Thus the ADA demonstrates a major ideological shift in the perception of disability. The commitment has changed from fixing and curing to accommodating and modifying.

This act is an important tool for parents. It allows for educational adaptations, modifications, and supports without the intensity of a full IEP.

SECTION 504 OF THE REHABILITATION ACT OF 1973
Some Frequently Asked Questions

1. What is a 504?

Section 504 of the Rehabilitation Act of 1973, Public Law 93-112 is a comprehensive law that addresses the rights of handicapped ("disabled") persons and applies to all agencies receiving federal financial assistance. Eliminating barriers to education programs and services, increasing building accessibility, and establishing equitable employment practices are thoroughly and specifically addressed in Section 504 regulations. The section states, ". . . no otherwise qualified handicapped individual in the United States, as defined in section 7(6), shall, solely by reason of his/her handicap, be excluded from the participation in, be denied the benefits of, or be subject to discrimination under any program or activity receiving federal financial assistance." The regulation makes it clear that the failure to provide a "free appropriate public education" to a disabled student covered by Section 504 is discrimination that violates the Act.

2. **Who is responsible for the enforcement and investigation of compliance with Section 504?**

The Office for Civil Rights (OCR) is responsible. Federal financial assistance to a local school district is contingent upon compliance with this and all other civil rights laws. The OCR may determine that federal funds should be withheld from local school systems that are not in compliance with civil rights legislation.

3. **Who is covered under Section 504?**

In 1973, when the Rehabilitation Act was passed, *handicap* was the acceptable term for a mental or physical impairment. Today, *disability* is preferred and promoted. But either refers to a person who (1) has either one which substantially limits one or more major life activities, or (2) has a record of such an impairment, or (3) is regarded as having such an impairment. To qualify for protection under the law, the individual must have a physical/mental disability that substantially limits a major life activity such as caring for oneself, performing manual tasks, walking, seeing, hearing, speaking, breathing, *learning,* and working. Examples include Tourette's syndrome, epilepsy, sickle-cell anemia, asthma, serious illness, or injury.

ADD/ADHD

When a school is informed that a student has attention deficit disorder (ADD) or attention deficit hyperactivity disorder (ADHD), the school is required to make appropriate accommodations for educating the student. These strategies can be documented on the Student Support Team Strategies/Minutes form or a similar type of recording instrument. Each school in the public sector must have in place a form for recording a child's weaknesses and strengths. For example, if inappropriate behavior is the manifestation of the student's condition, then the successful development of a behavior management plan meets the school's obligations under federal law.

If the student is manifesting attention problems that are affecting learning, the Student Support Team (SST) (usually includes the principal or vice principal, resource teacher, school counselor/psychologist, and classroom teacher) can develop strategies to address those within the regular classroom using the SST . When ADD results in behavior or attention problems so severe that they cannot be regularly accommodated, the school is obligated under Section 504 to provide special services to enable the student to benefit from an educational program. Students may qualify under IDEA as a student suffering from an "other health impairment (OHI)." The SST should then determine if it needs to make a referral to special education for consideration of OHI eligibility.

4. Who determines if a student is eligible for a 504?

Referrals begin at the local school level and are made to the SST. The SST process should be followed:

1. Initiate services

2. Clarify disability and needs

3. Generate a 504 accommodation plan

4. Evaluate plan

5. Monitor

6. Reevaluate

5. How does the student support team determine if a student is 504 eligible?

To qualify for protection under Section 504, the individual must have a physical or mental impairment that substantially limits a major life activity such as caring for oneself, performing manual tasks, walking, seeing, hearing, speaking, breathing, learning, or working. Three questions to consider in determining whether a person's impairment substantially limits one or more major life activities are (1) What is the nature and severity of the impairment? (2) How long will it last or is it expected to last? and (3) What is its permanent or long-term impact or expected impact? Temporary, nonchronic impairments that do not last for a long time and that have little or no long-term impact usually are not considered to be disabilities.

6. What is a section 504 accommodation plan?

Although a written plan is not required in federal regulations, it is advised and practical; it makes good sense that the plan be in writing. Parents should be notified and parental rights given. See Appendix C.

7. Where are parents' rights under section 504?

See Appendix D.

8. What are reasonable accommodations?

Reasonable accommodations in the school setting are modifications or adjustments of educational programs to afford students with disabilities equal opportunity to access the programs. Schools must provide reasonable accommodations to students with disabilities unless schools can show that the requested accommodations would impose undue hardship. The concept of undue hardship includes any action that is unduly costly, extensive, substantial, or disruptive, or would fundamentally alter the nature of operation of the program. Accommodations include extended time for test/projects/assignments and all items listed on the psychoeducational evaluation.

9. What are some examples of classroom and facility accommodations?

Refer to Appendix E for accommodations in the areas of communication, organization management, alternative teaching strategies, and student precautions.

10. What are the guidelines for special test accommodations under section 504?

An accommodation plan must be on file for each student for whom modifications will be made. The plan should outline instructional modifications appropriate for the student during regular classroom instruction. Testing modifications consistent with other instructional modifications should also be outlined in the plan. It is not appropriate to make testing modifications unless the appropriate documentation is on file. Students who are tested under Section 504 guidelines and receive modification on the Iowa Test of Basic Skills (ITBS) may be coded 99. Modifications made on some norm-referenced tests might invalidate the results.

Notes

No. 10: *This is our major concern!*

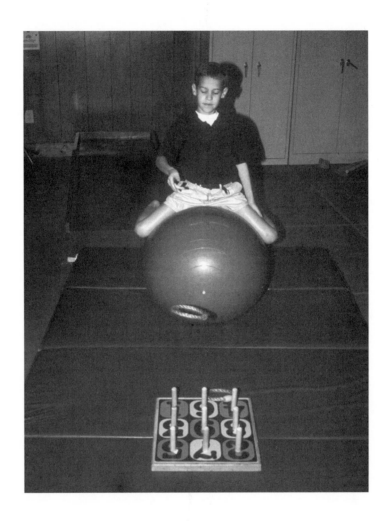

APPENDIX C

Section 504 Student Accommodation Plan

SECTION 504

STUDENT ACCOMMODATION PLAN

I. Name: _____ II. DOB: _____/_____/_____

III. School: _____ Grade: _____

IV. Date of meeting: _____

V. Describe the disabling condition: _____

_____

_____

_____

_____

VI. Describe how the disability affects a major life activity: _____

_____

Educational impact: _____

_____

VII. Describe the reasonable accommodations that are necessary: _____

_____

_____

_____

_____

VIII. Location of accommodations: ( ) Regular class   ( ) Other

IX. Review / Reassessment date: _____

X. Participant's name: Title: Date:

_____   _____   _____

_____   _____   _____

_____   _____   _____

XI. I have participated in the development of this plan and have received a copy of the Notice of Section 504 Rights.

Parent signature: _____ Date: _____

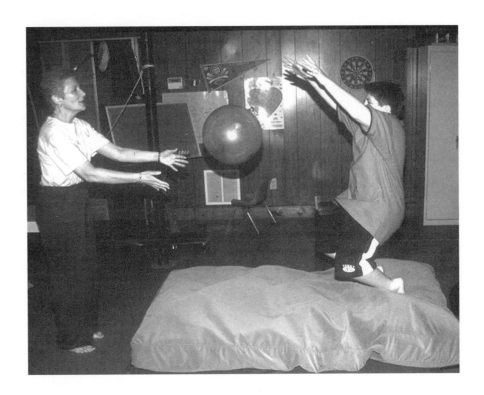

APPENDIX D

Section 504 Parent Rights

Section 504 Parent Rights

1. Right to file a grievance with the school district over an alleged violation of Section 504 regulations.
2. Right to have an evaluation that draws on information from a variety of sources.
3. Right to have program/service decisions made by a group of persons who know the needs of the student, the meaning of evaluation data, and program/service options.
4. Right to be informed of any proposed actions related to eligibility and plan for services.
5. Right to examine all relevant records.
6. Right to receive all information in the parents'/guardians' native language and primary mode of communication.
7. If the student is eligible under Section 504, the right to periodic reevaluations and an evaluation before any significant change in program/service modifications.
8. Right to an impartial hearing if there is a disagreement with the school district's proposed action.
9. Right to be represented by counsel in the impartial hearing process.
10. Right to appeal the impartial hearing officer's decision.

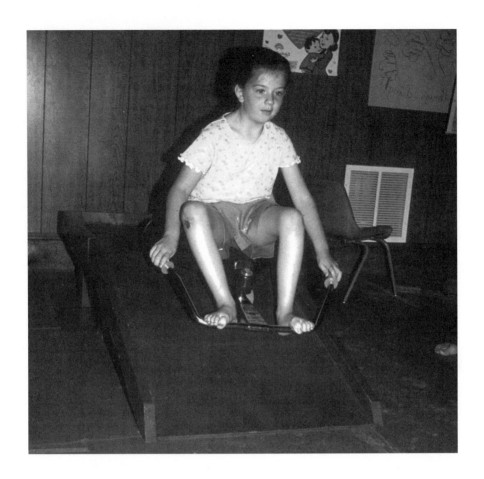

APPENDIX E

Classroom and Facility Accommodations

As local districts develop policies and procedures for guiding the referral and identification of students determined to be handicapped under Section 504, it is critical that information concerning this law and its impact on local school districts be shared with principals and building-level staff. The intent of Section 504 is to accommodate for differences within the regular education environment. For this to be accomplished, all staff must be provided with awareness activities and be given specific information concerning the district's procedures for dealing with Section 504 referrals.

As individual students are identified, the classroom teacher may need specific training in the area of the identified handicap (e.g., training from the school nurse on danger signs of an impending asthma attack, training from a physical therapist on correct positioning of a wheelchair-bound student at his or her desk, etc.). The following classroom facility accommodations are presented as examples of ways in which Section 504 handicaps may be successfully addressed within the regular education environment.

I. Communication

   A. There may be a need to modify parent/student/teacher communications

      1. Develop a daily/weekly journal

      2. Develop parent/student/school contacts

      3. Schedule periodic parent/teacher meetings

   B. There may be a need to modify staff communications

      1. Identify resource staff for extended time testing as needed

      2. Network with other staff

      3. Schedule building-level team meetings

      4. Maintain on-going communication with building principal

   C. There may be a need to modify school/community agency communication. With parent consent:

      1. Identify and communicate with appropriate agency personnel working with student

2. Assist in agency referrals

3. Provide appropriate carry-over in the school environment

II. Organization/Management

A. There may be a need to modify the instructional day

1. Allow student more time to pass in hallways

2. Modify class schedule

B. There may be a need to modify the classroom organization/structure

1. Adjust placement of student within classroom (e.g., study carrel, proximity to teacher, etc.)

2. Increase/Decrease opportunity for movement

3. Determine appropriate classroom assignment (i.e., open versus structured)

4. Reduce external stimuli

C. There may be a need to modify the district's policies/procedures

1. Allow increase in number of excused absences for health reasons

2. Adjust transportation/parking arrangements

3. Approve early dismissal for service agency appointments

III. Alternative Teaching Strategies

A. There may be a need to modify teaching methods

1. Adjust testing procedures (e.g., length of time, oral administration, tape recorded answers, etc.)

2. Utilize materials that address the student's learning style (e.g., visual, tactile, auditory, etc.)

3. Adjust reading level of materials

IV. Student Precautions

A. There may be a need to modify the classroom/building climate for health purposes

1. Use an air purifier in classroom

2. Control temperature

3. Accommodate specific allergic reactions

B. There may be a need to modify classroom/building to accommodate equipment needs

1. Plan for evaluation for wheelchair-bound students

2. Schedule classes in accessible areas

C. There may be a need to modify building health/safety procedures

1. Administer medication

2. Apply universal precautions

3. Accommodate special diet

Now—Go out and follow your own best advice!

Susan N. Schriber Orloff, OTR/L
